Mandalas for Mindfulness
Volume 1

31 Mandalas & Inspirational Quotes

Adult Coloring Book for Relief from Stress,
Anxiety & Depression

By Nerine Martin
ColorYourWayToHappy.com

Cover and Book Design by Nerine Martin

www.ColorYourWayToHappy.com

Preview of Designs Inside this Book

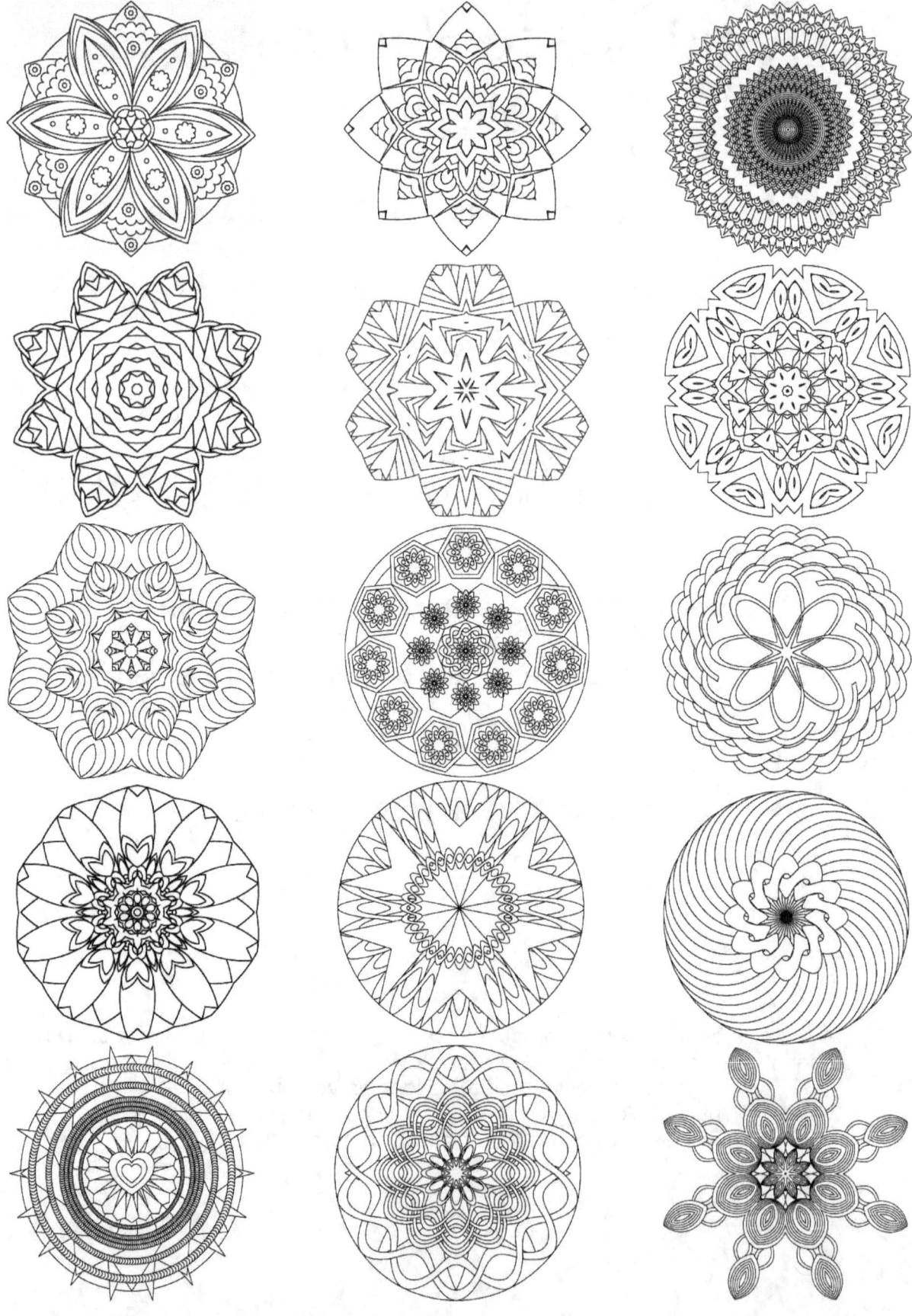

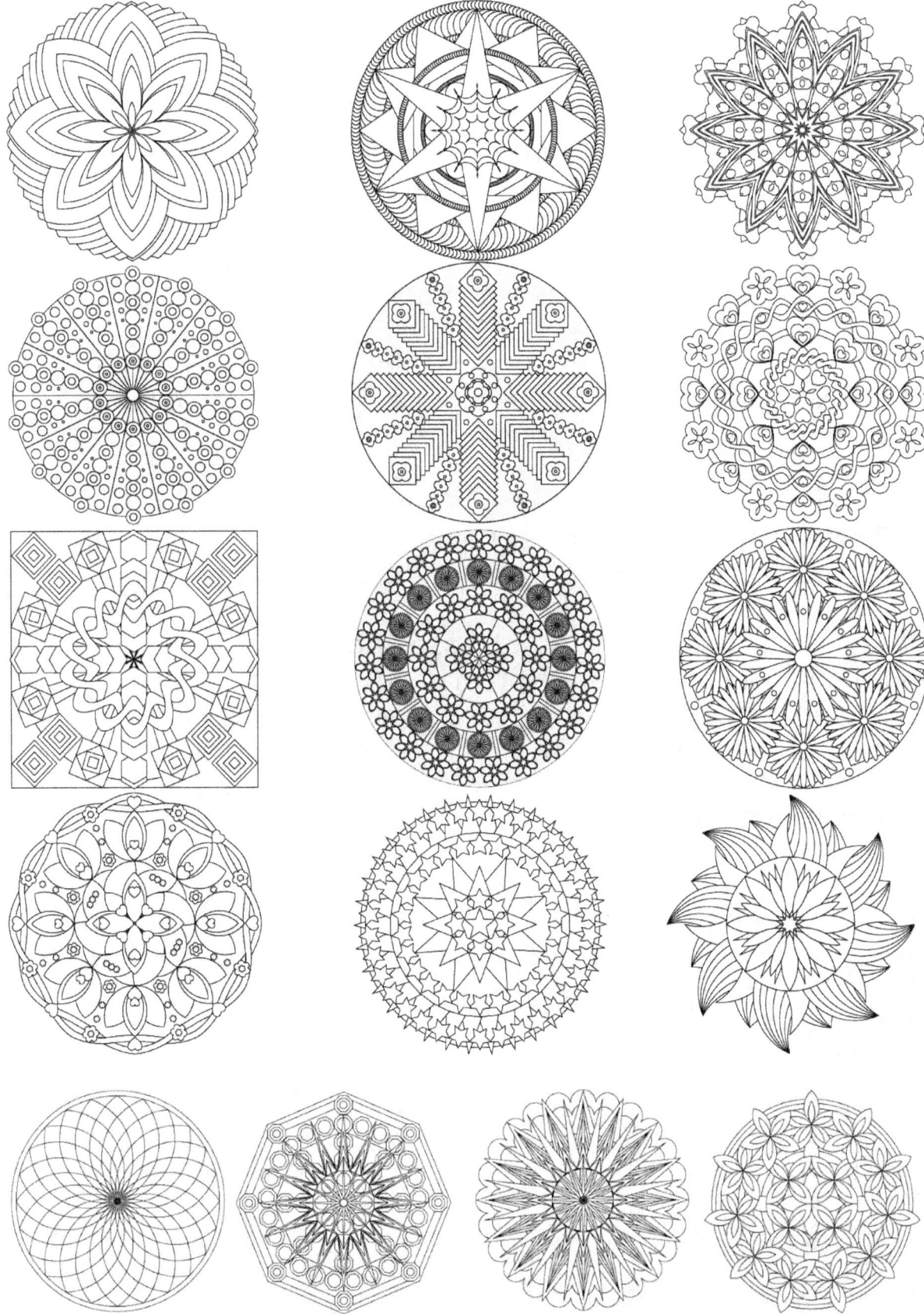

Congratulations on your purchase of *Mandalas for Mindfulness Volume 1* and thank you for choosing my coloring book.

This coloring book is suitable for colorers of all levels and with 31 single sided printed mandalas, you can choose to color a new one every day of the month to help you de-stress and relax. There are also 31 inspirational quotes to help reinforce a positive mindset, while you enjoy your coloring experience.

Use your imagination to make these designs come alive with color, using colored pencils, felt tip markers, gel pens, fluoro markers, metallic pens or crayons.

To help prevent any bleed through when using felt tip markers – place a blank sheet of paper behind the page when coloring. You can find spare pages located at the back of this book.

Please remember that your purchase of this coloring book is for your personal use only and you may not share or copy the uncolored pages for others. Please direct other people to purchase their own copy. By doing so, you are supporting my art so I can continue to make more coloring books and I thank you for your understanding and support. ☺

I hope you enjoy coloring my book and that you 'Color Your Way To Happy'.

Yours in coloring,

Nerine ☺

P.S. If you enjoy this coloring book, please be so kind to leave a review on Amazon.

Use This Area To Test Your Colors

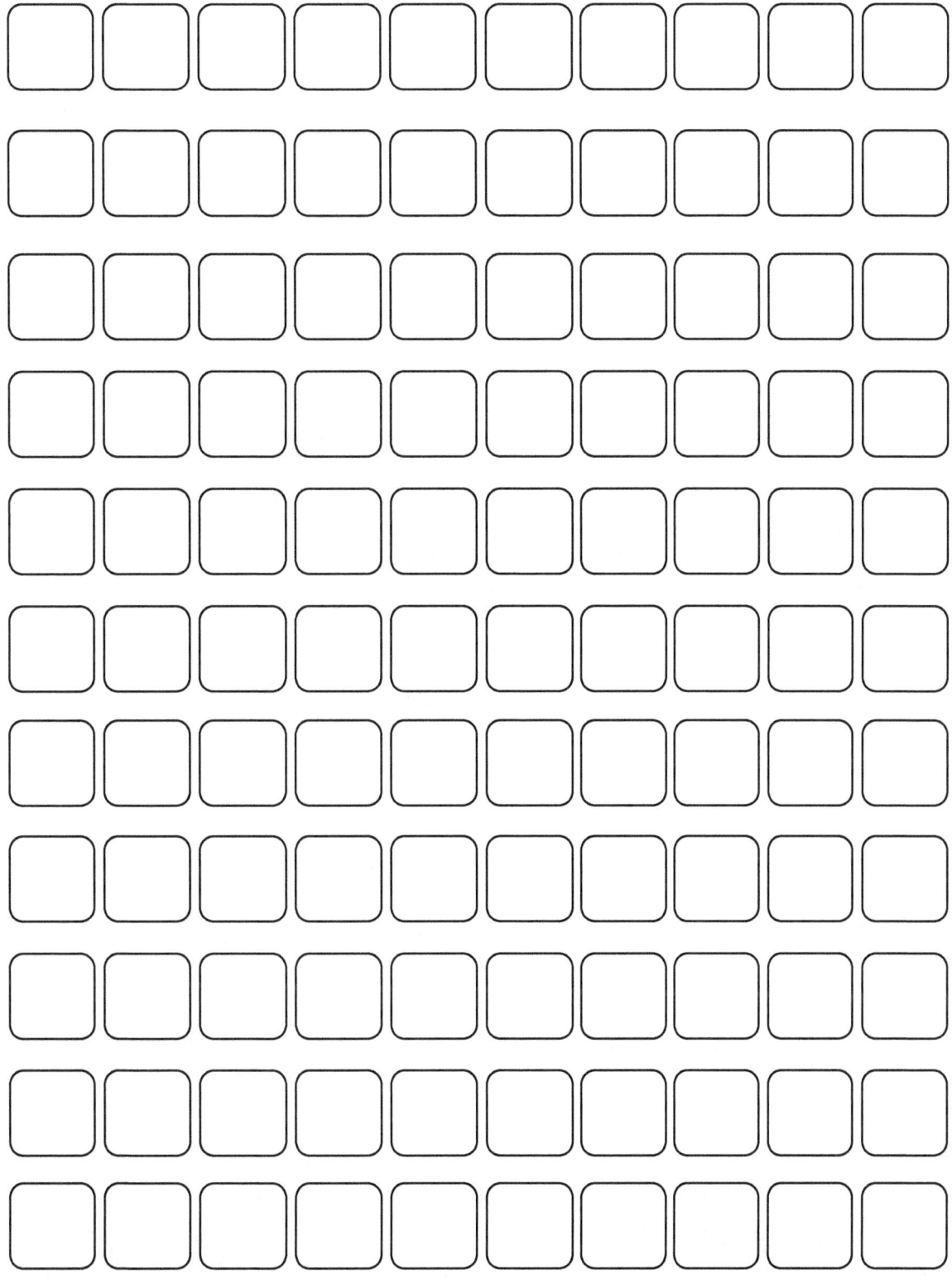

"If you can dream it, then
you can achieve it."

Zig Ziglar

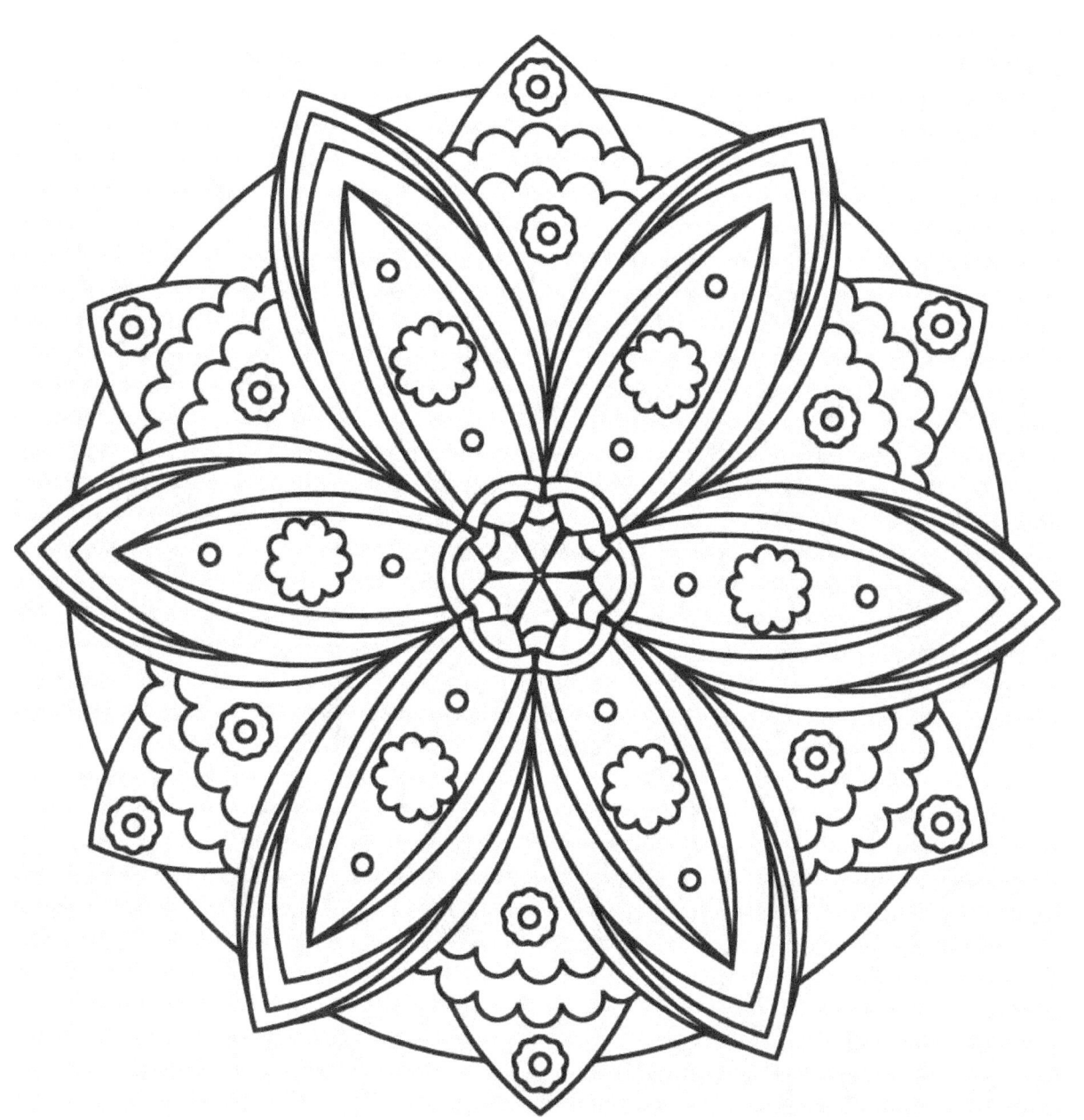

I am in control of my thoughts!

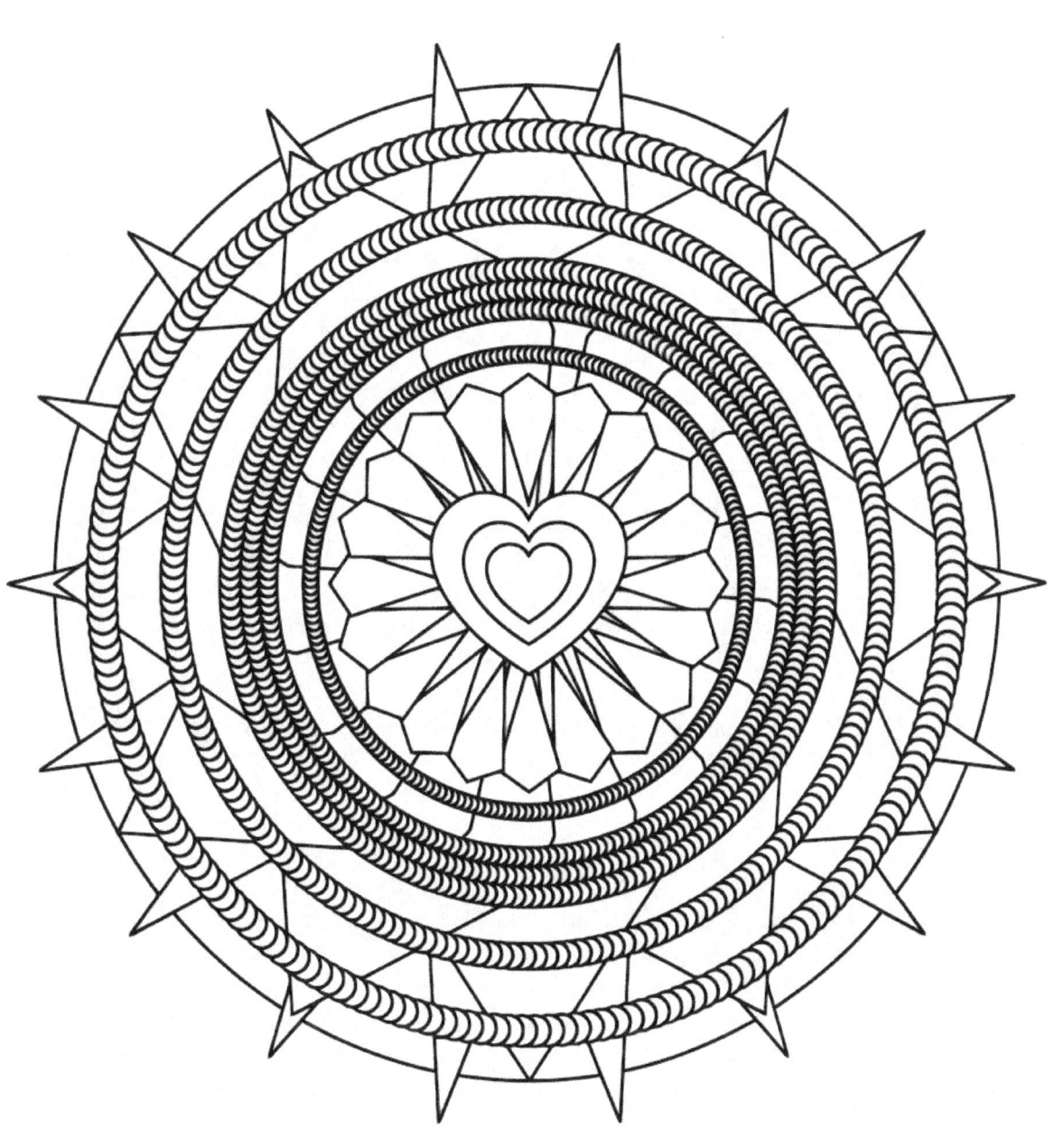

*Happiness is a new
coloring book!*

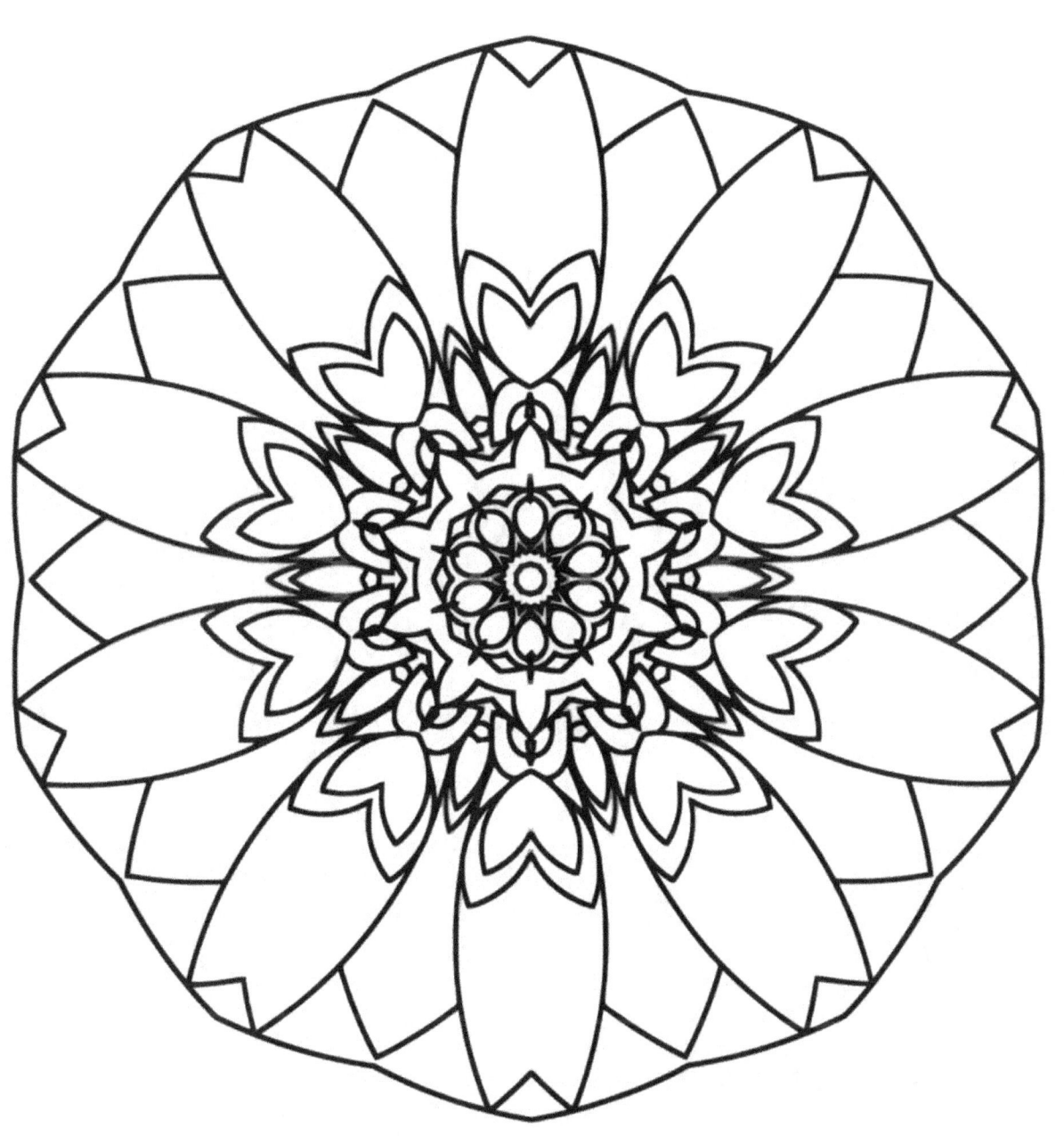

"FEAR has two meanings:
'Forget everything and
run' or
'Face everything and rise'
The choice is yours!"

Zig Ziglar

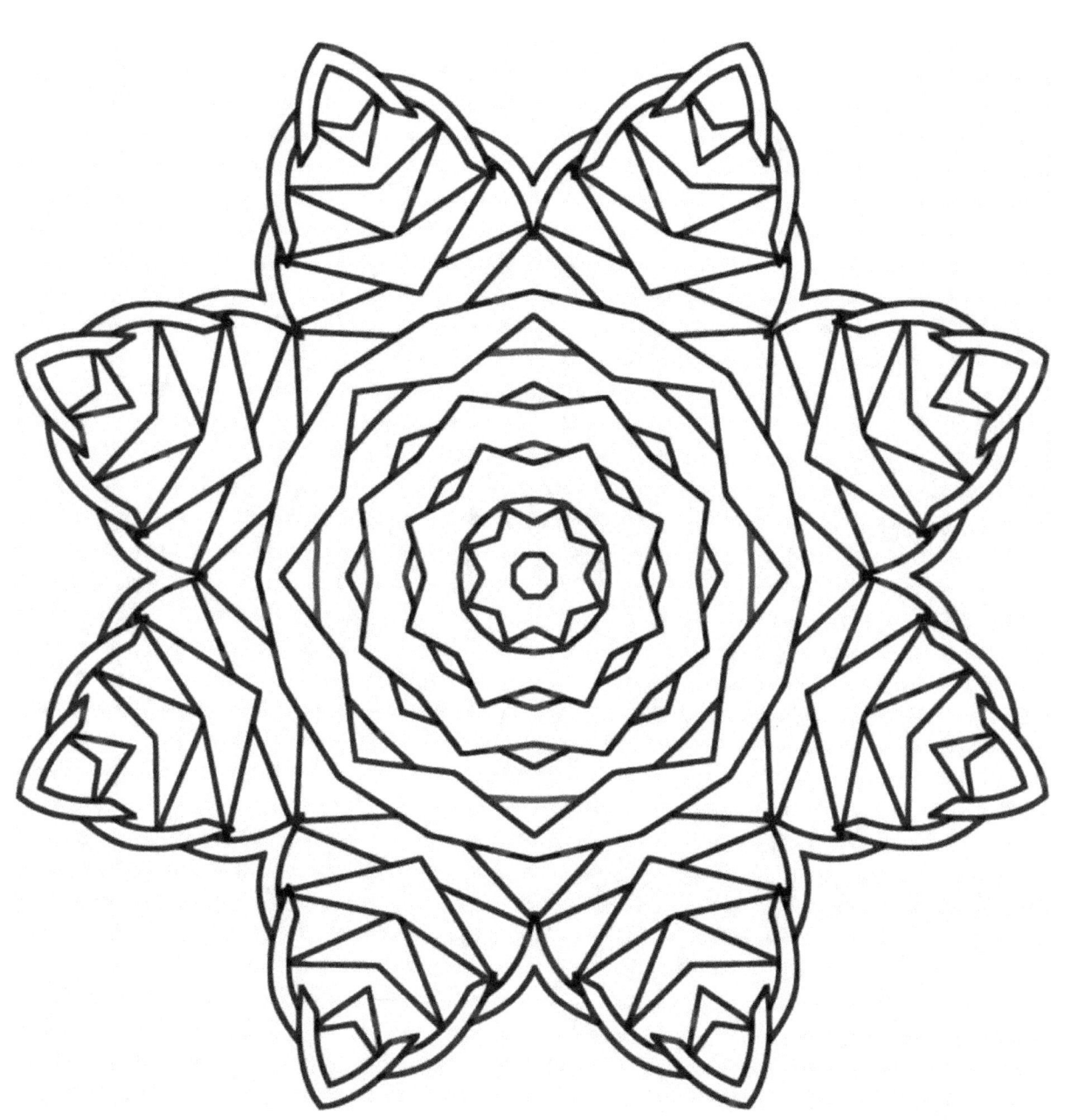

*Always believe that
something wonderful
is about to happen.*

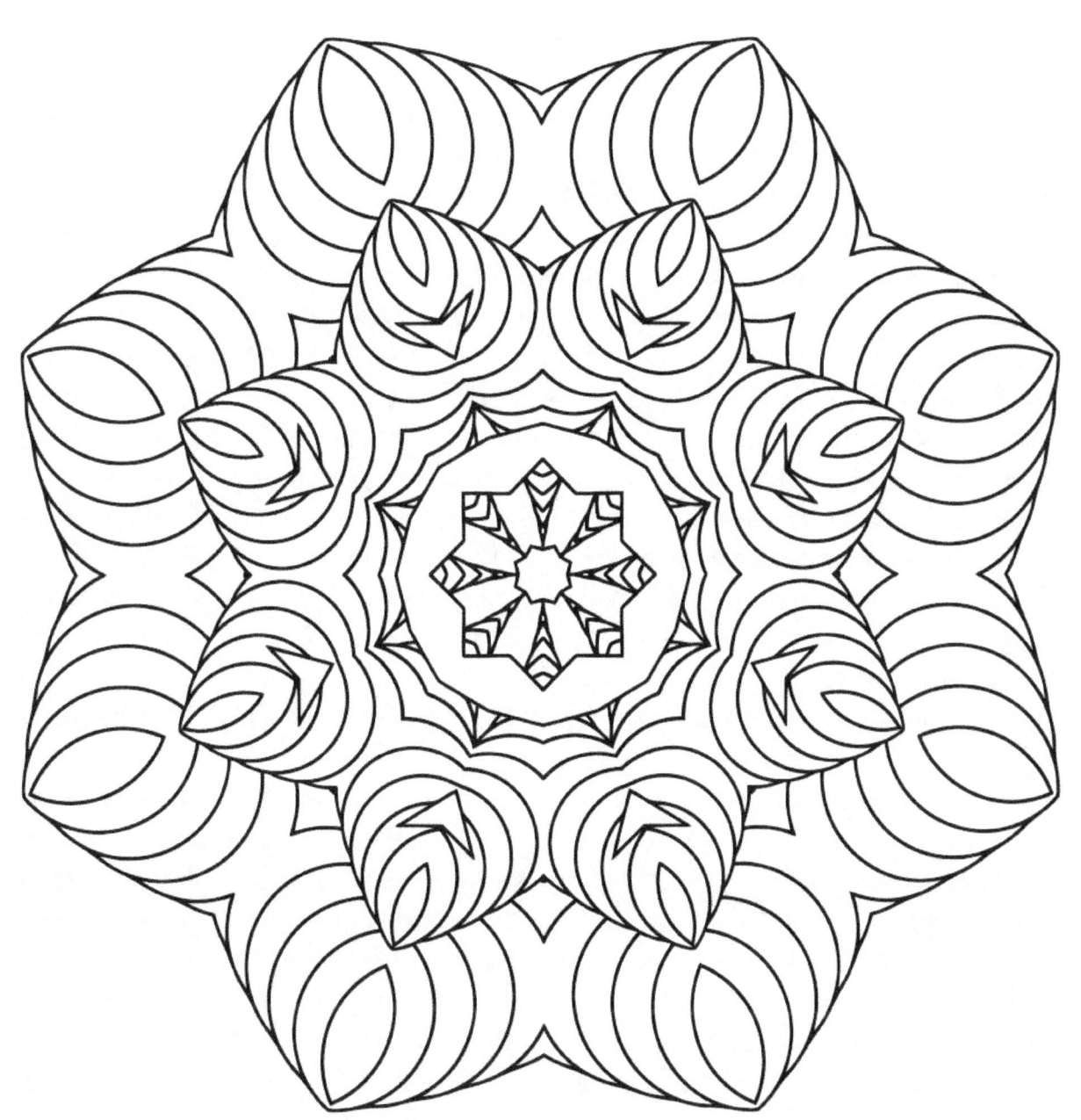

*Do more of what makes
you happy!*

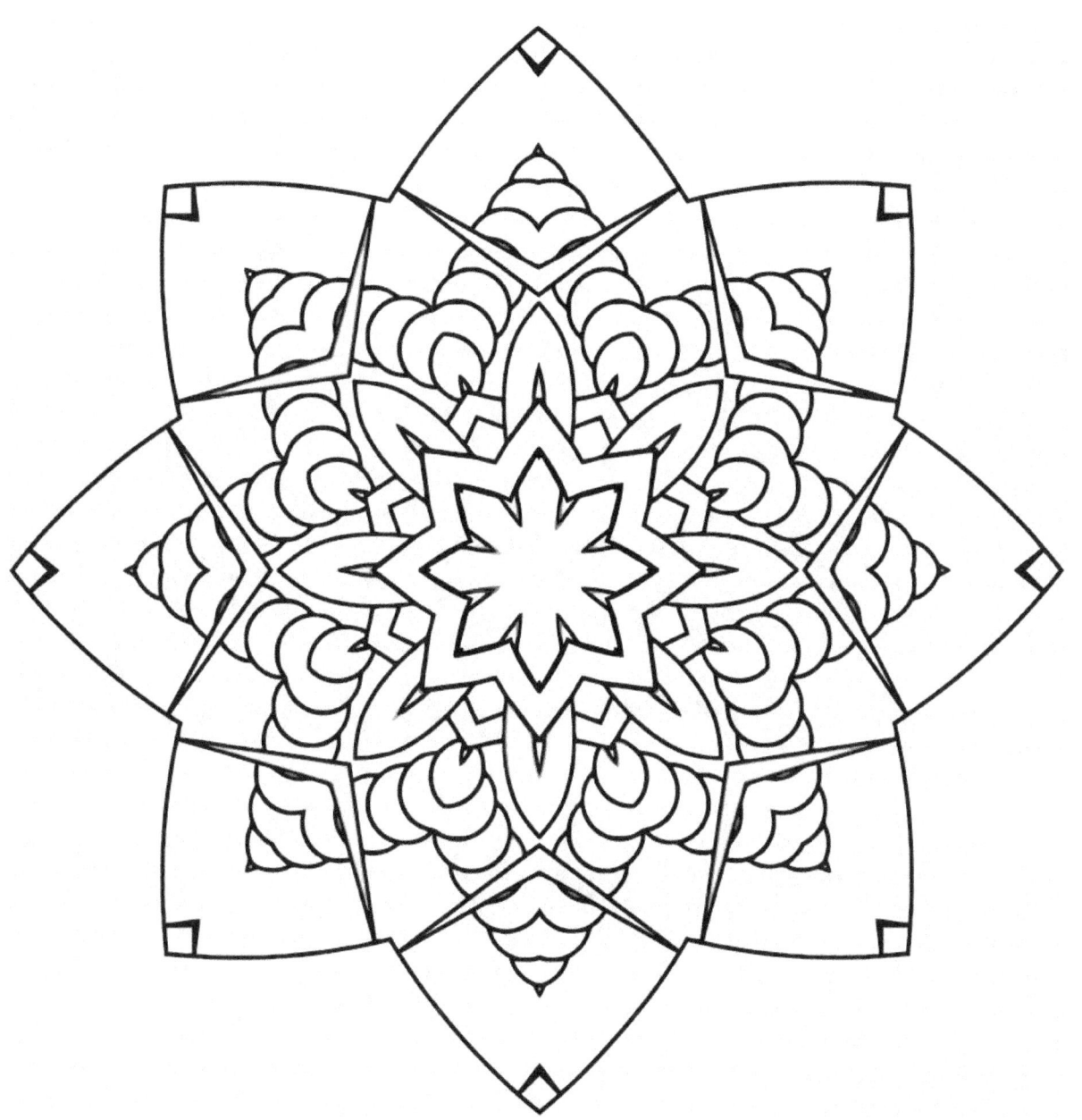

Focus on the good in your life!

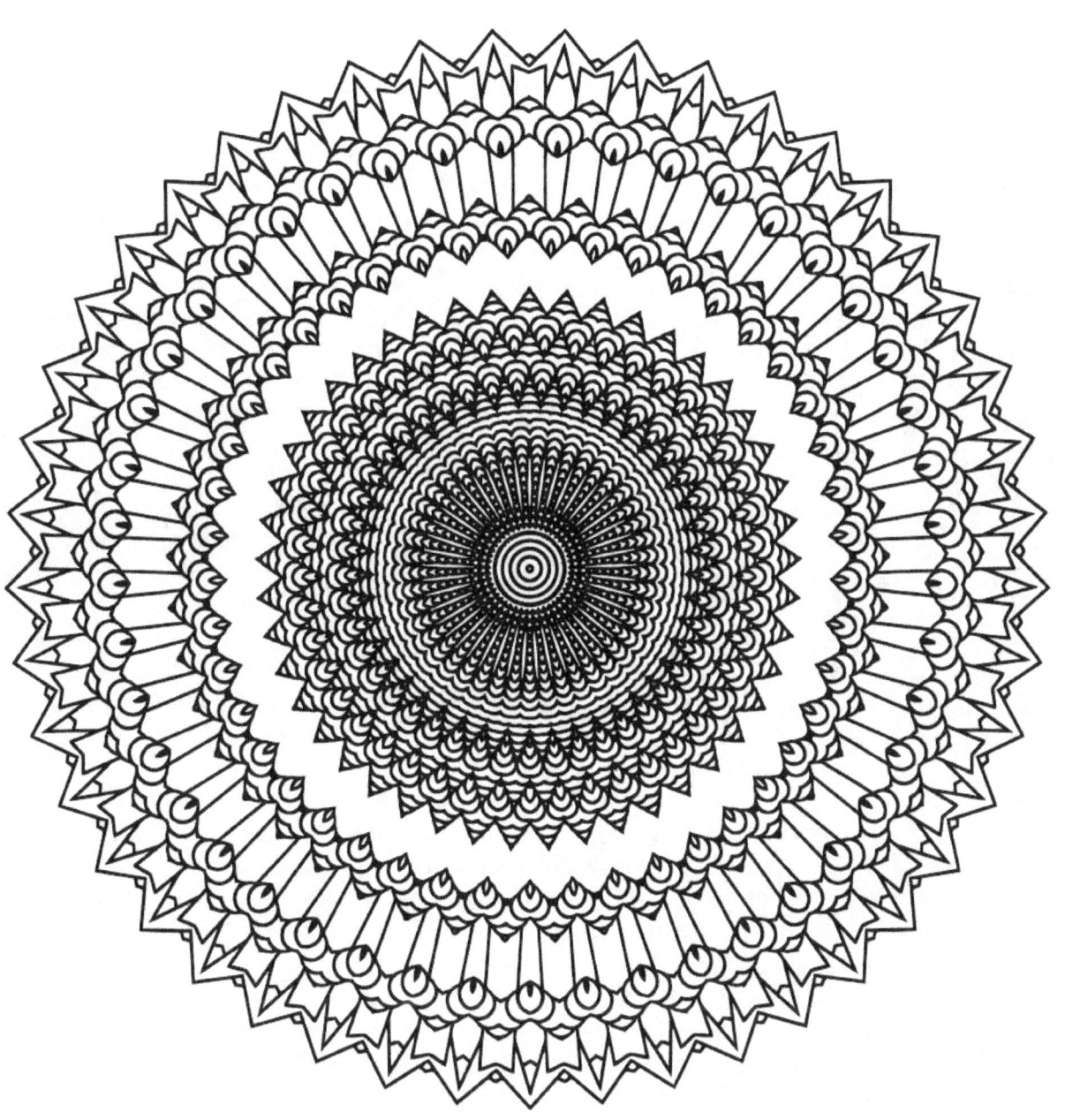

"We cannot start over,
but we can begin now and
make a new ending."

Zig Ziglar

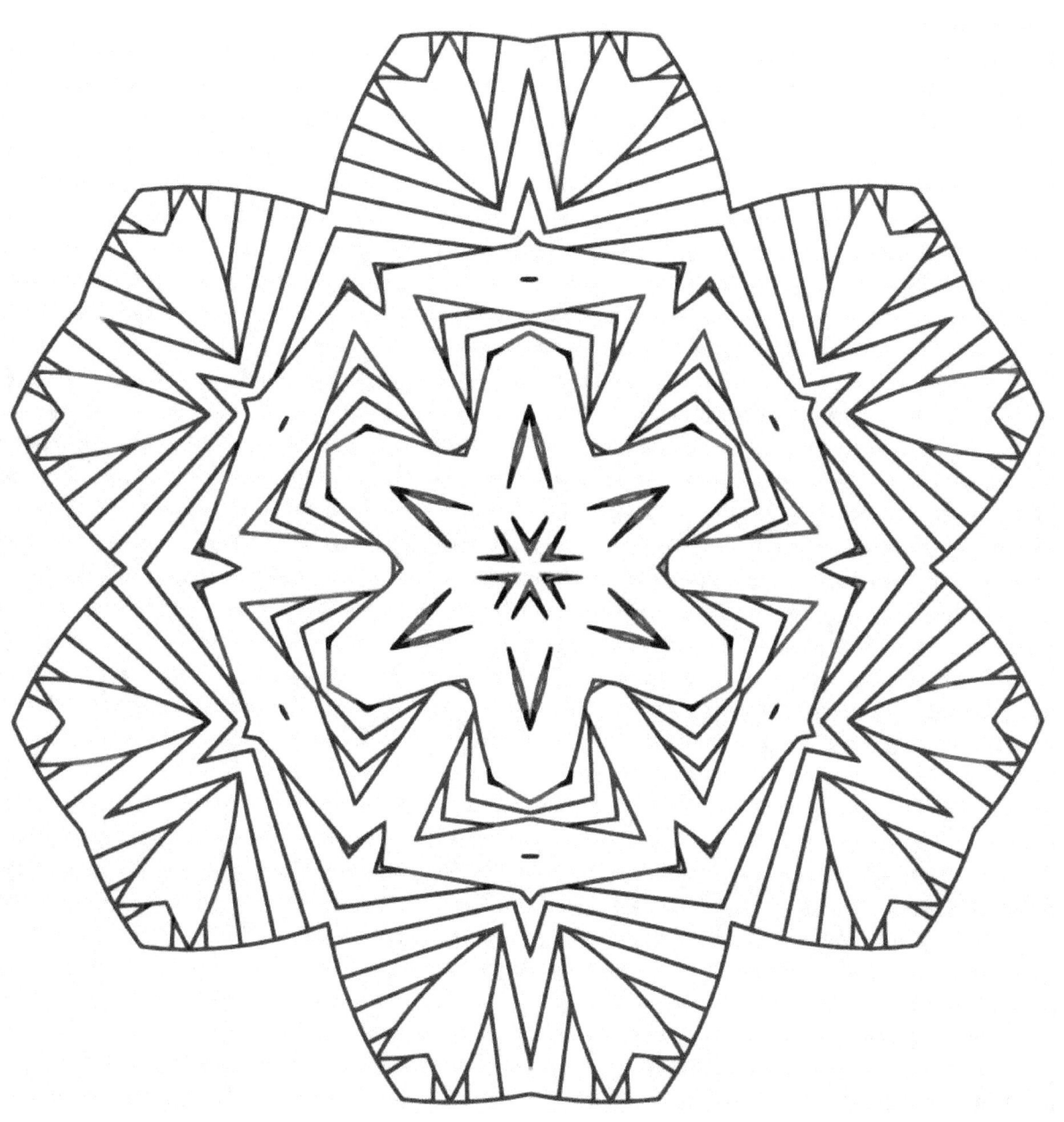

Worrying won't stop the bad stuff from happening, it just stops you from enjoying the good.

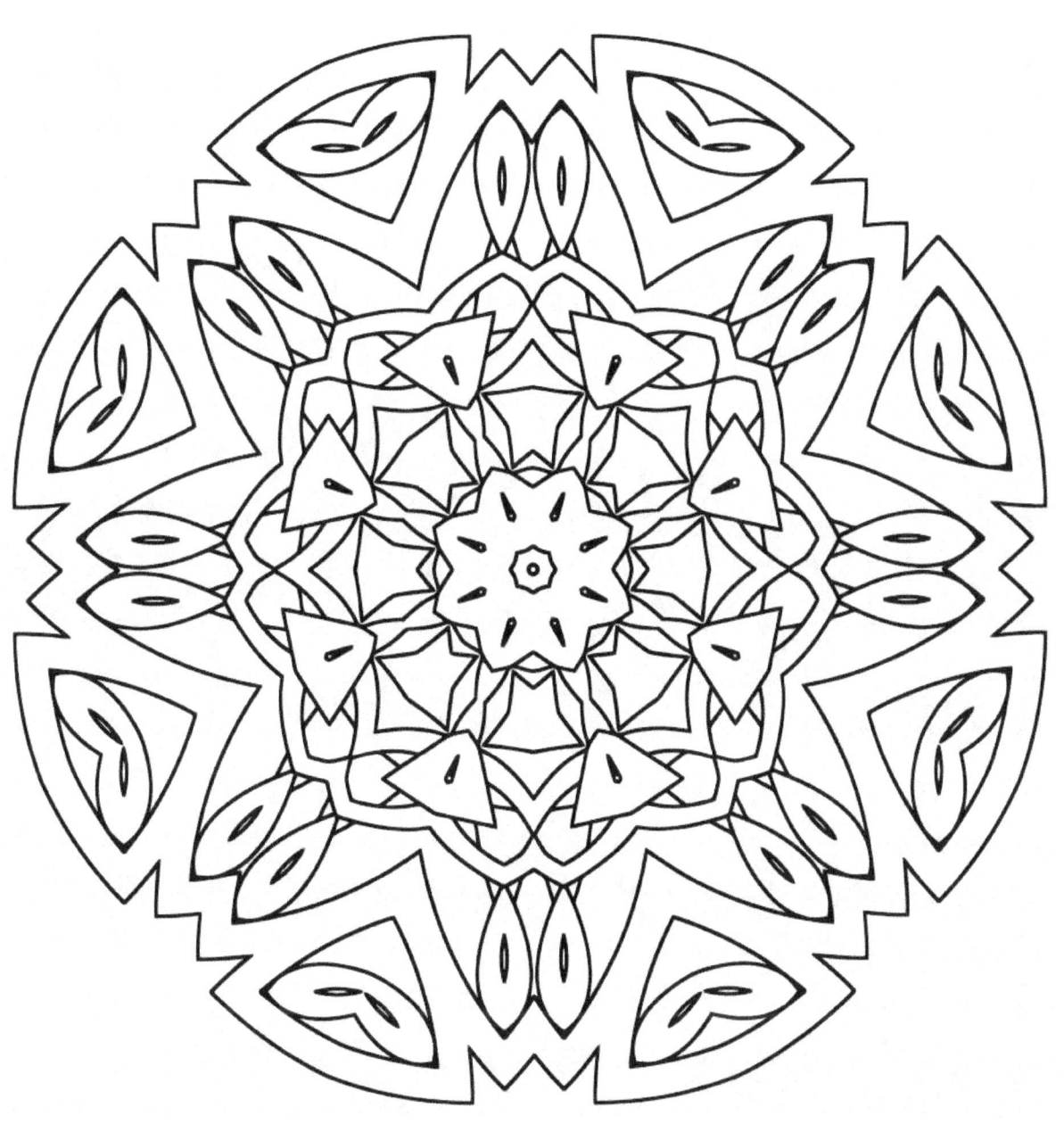

Color like nobody is watching!

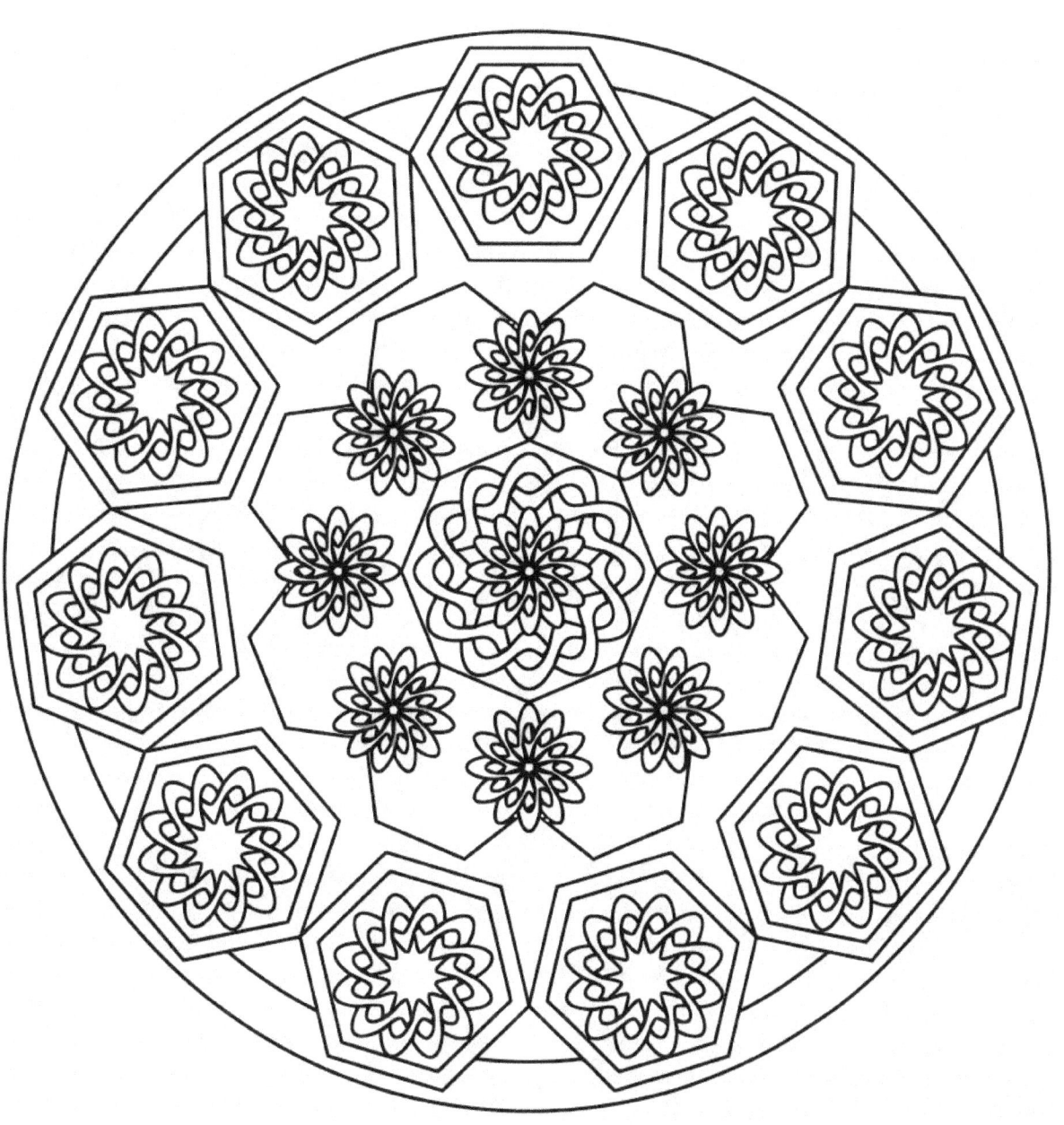

You are good enough!

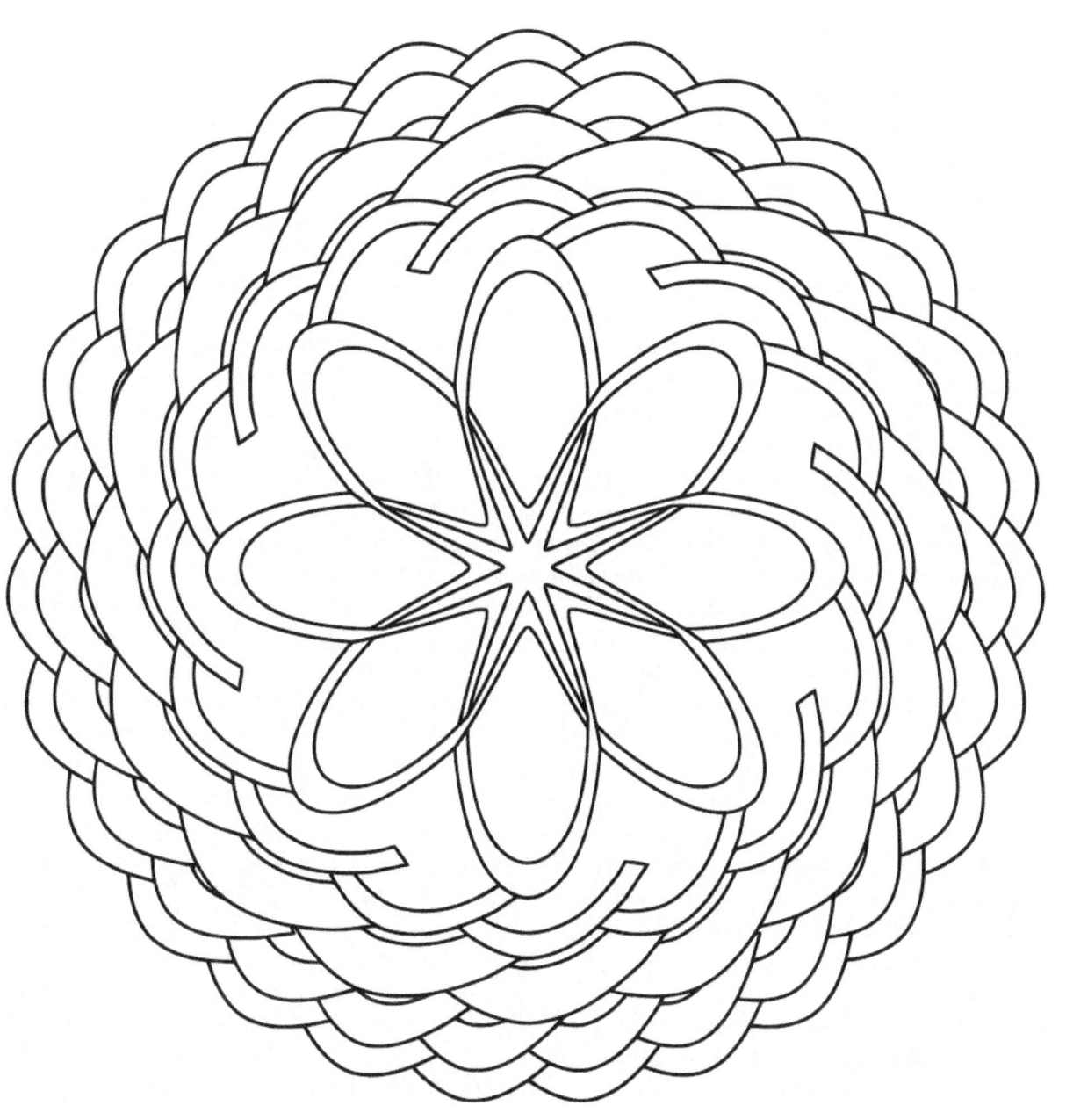

Life is better when you're laughing!

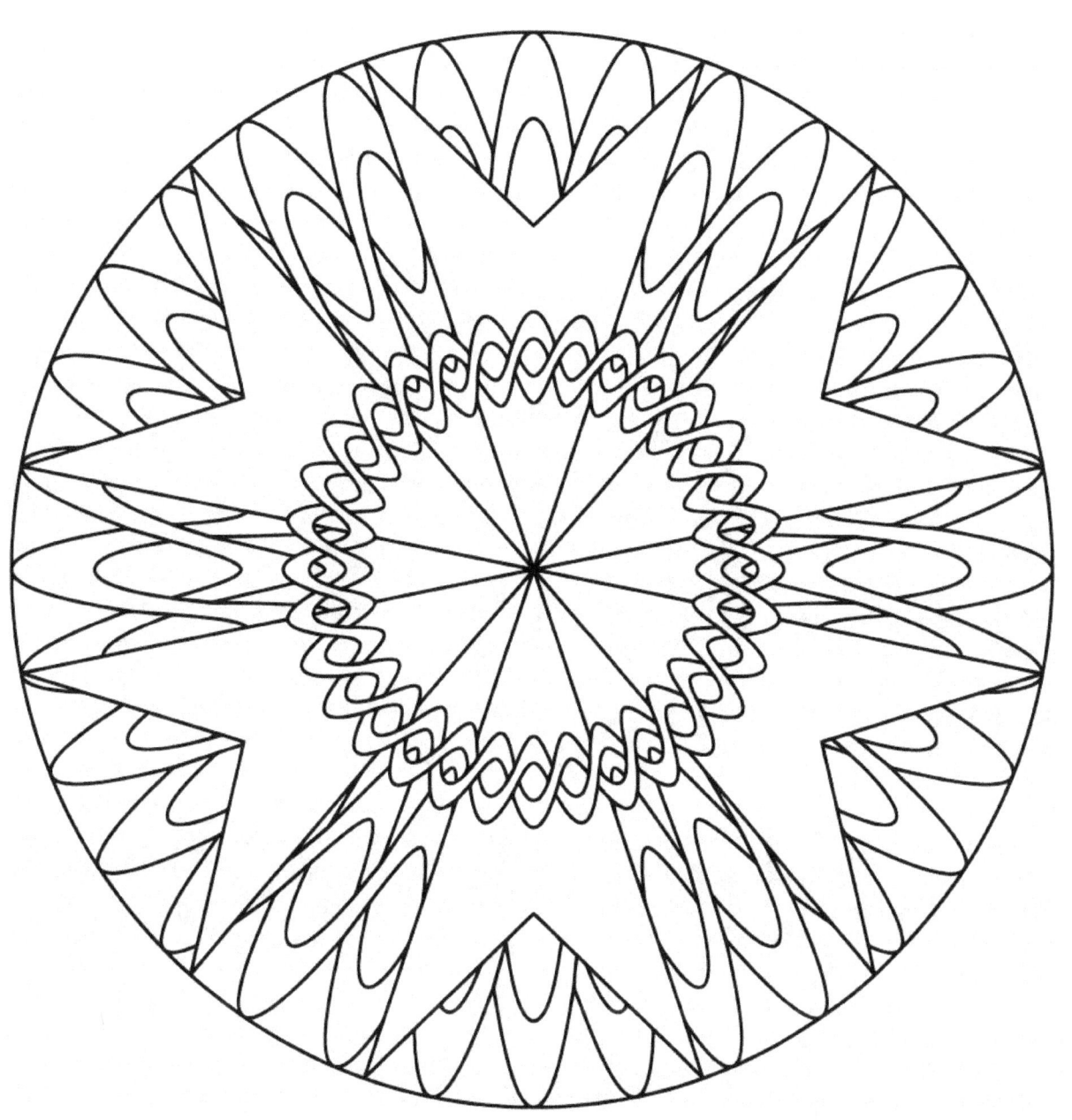

*Some days you have to
create your own sunshine!*

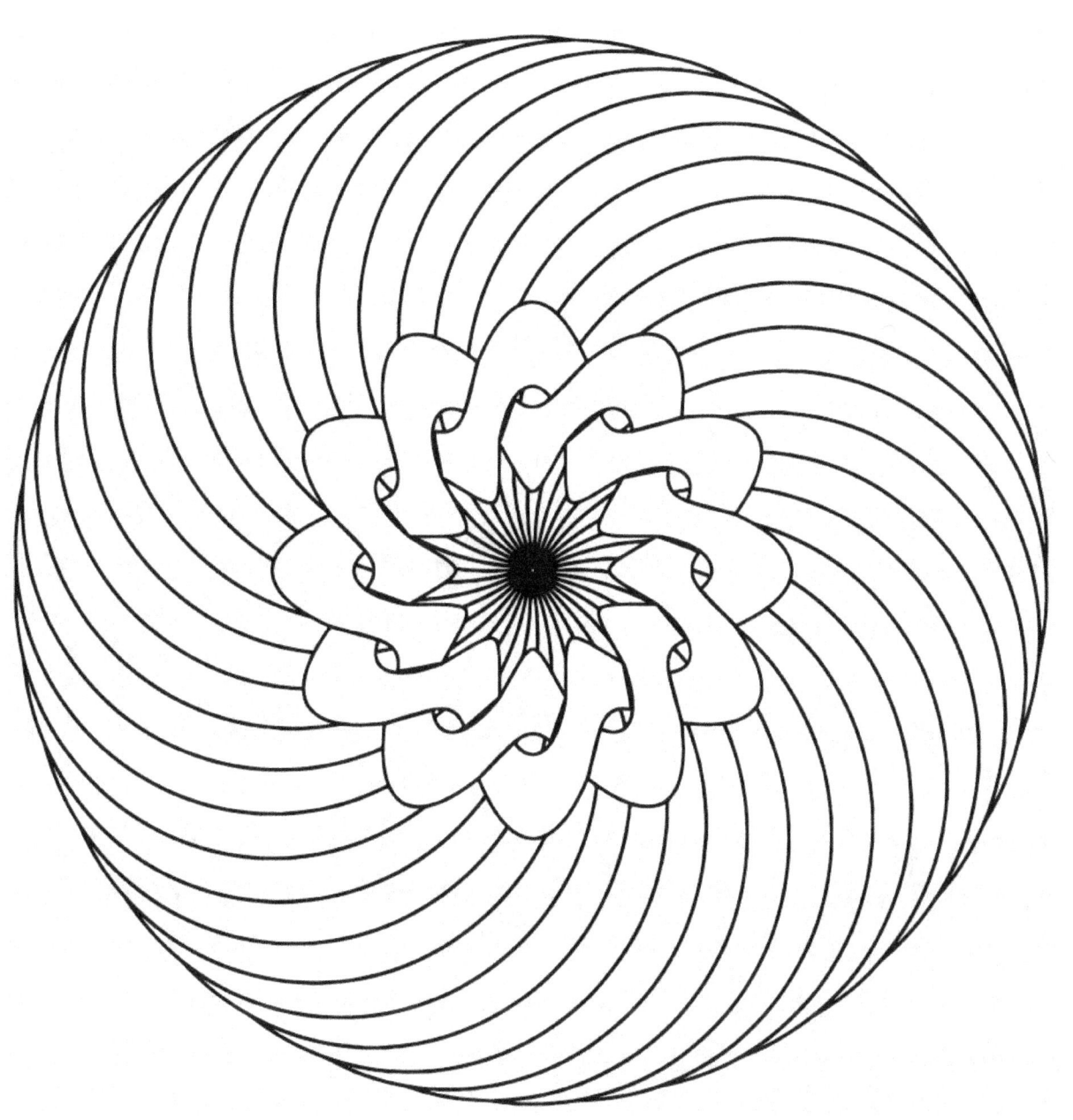

Enjoy the moment!

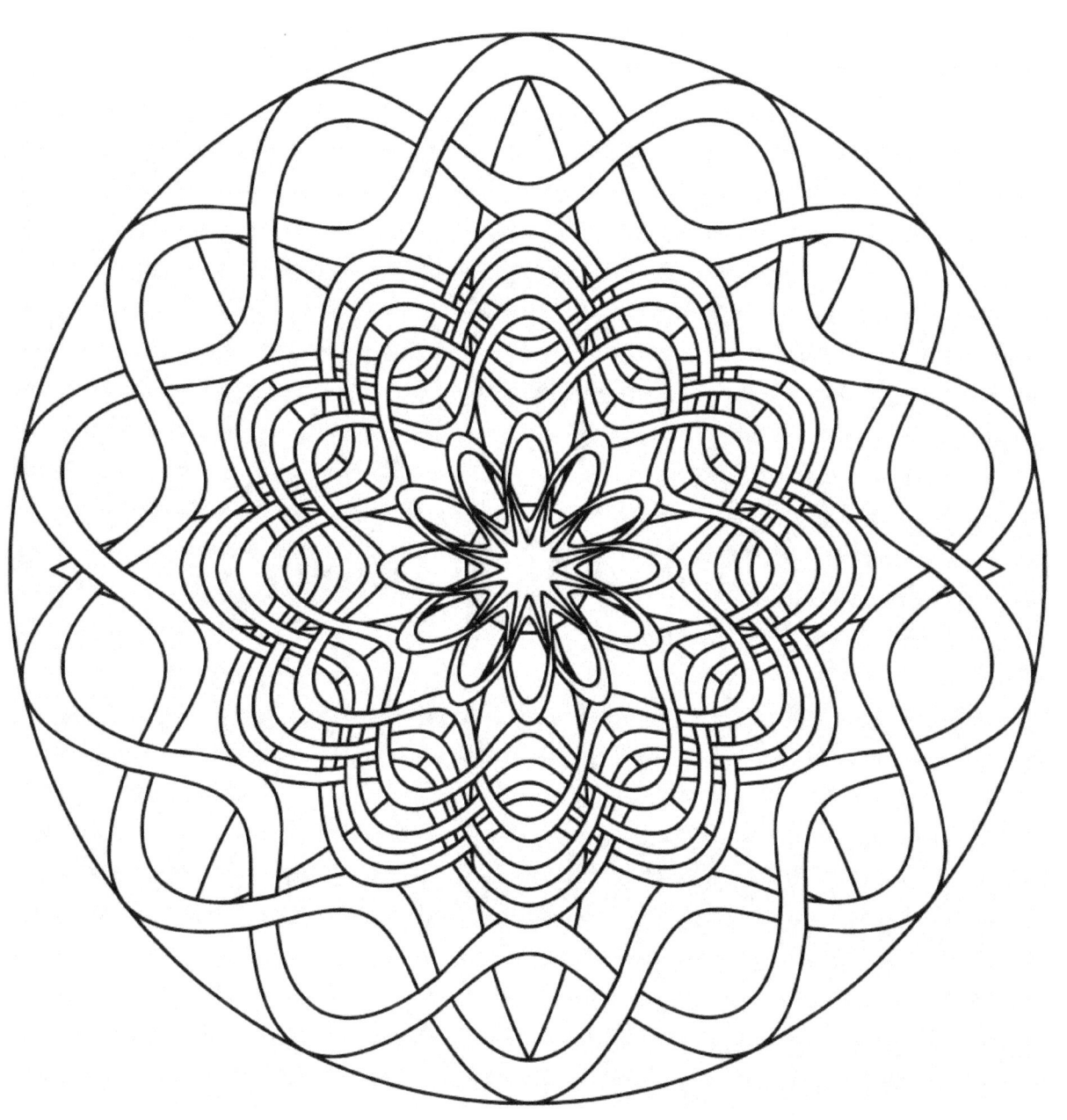

Do what you love, often!

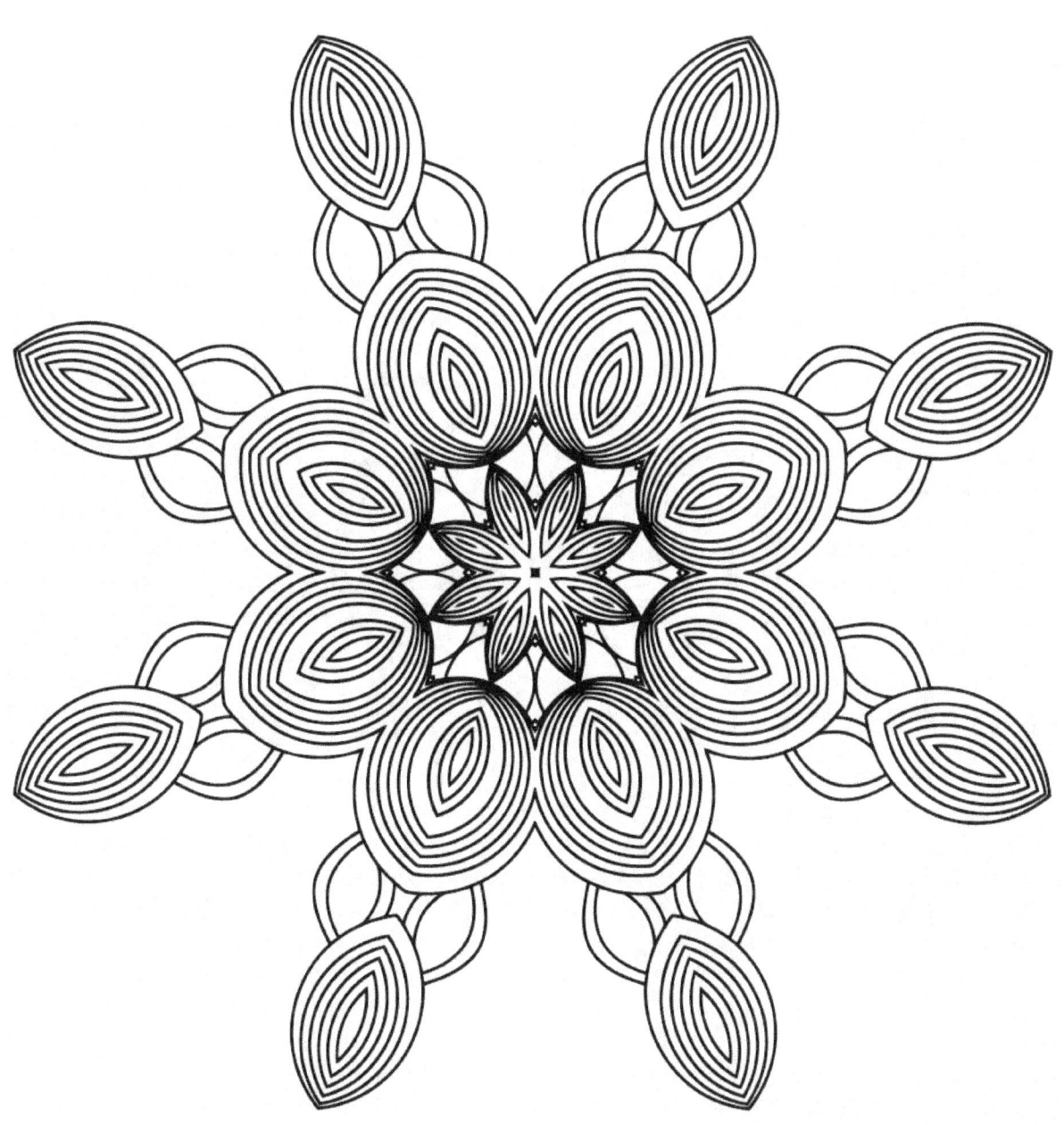

*"What you get by
achieving your goals is
not as important
as what you become by
achieving your goals."*

Zig Ziglar

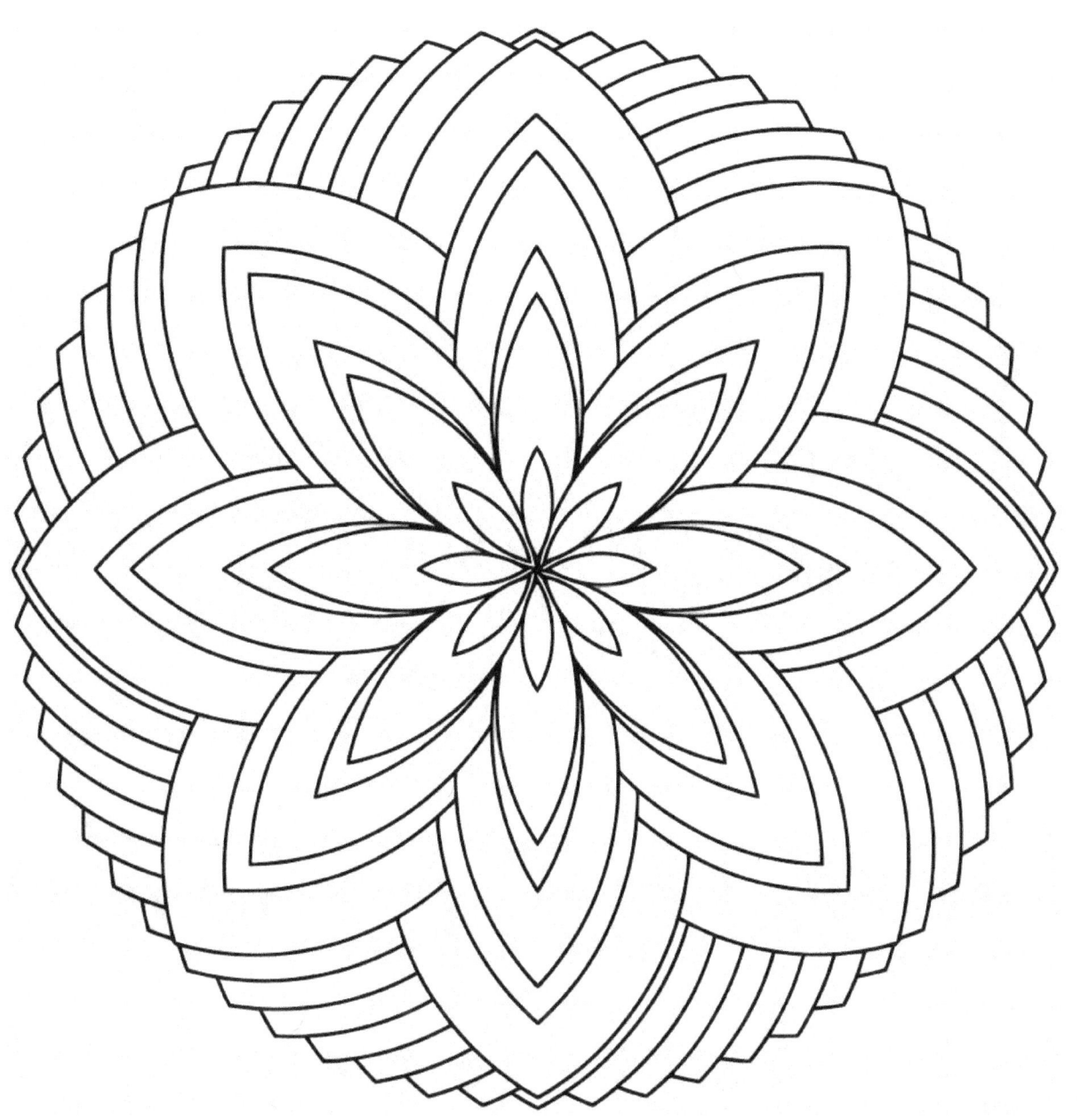

We either make ourselves
miserable
or we make ourselves
strong.
The amount of work is the
same.

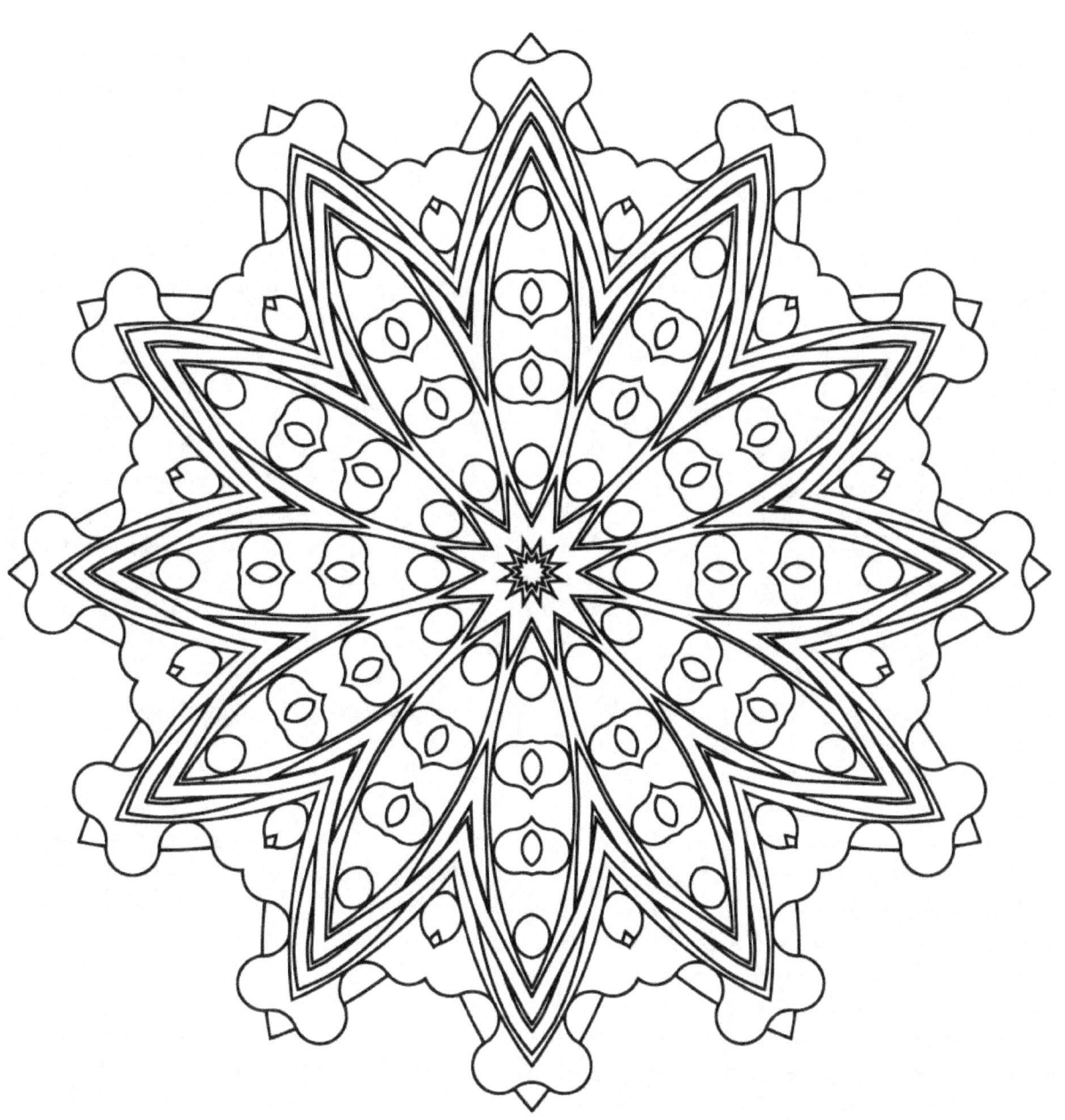

*You are beautiful inside
and out!*

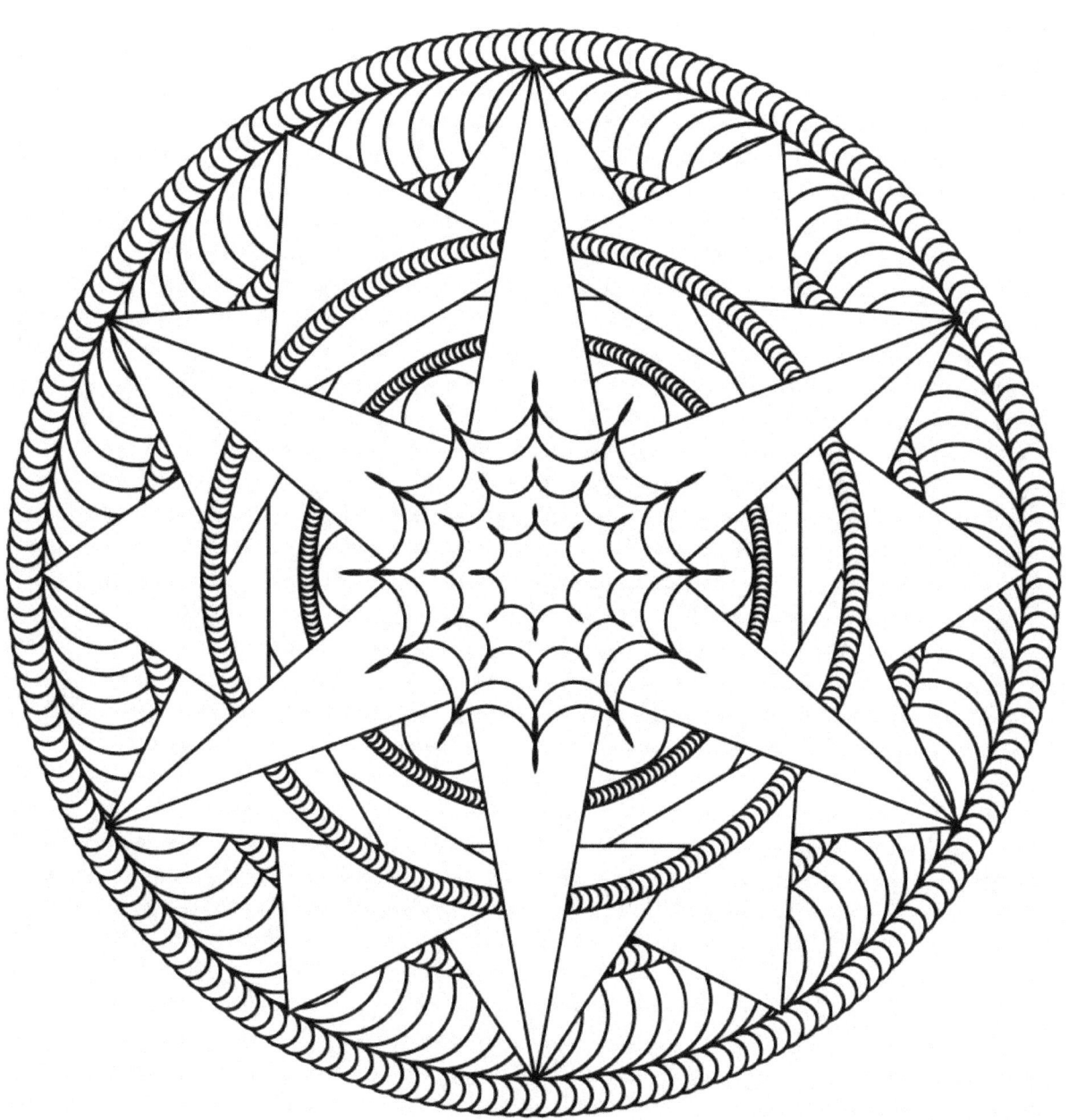

"People often say motivation doesn't last. Neither does bathing - that's why we recommend it daily."

Zig Ziglar

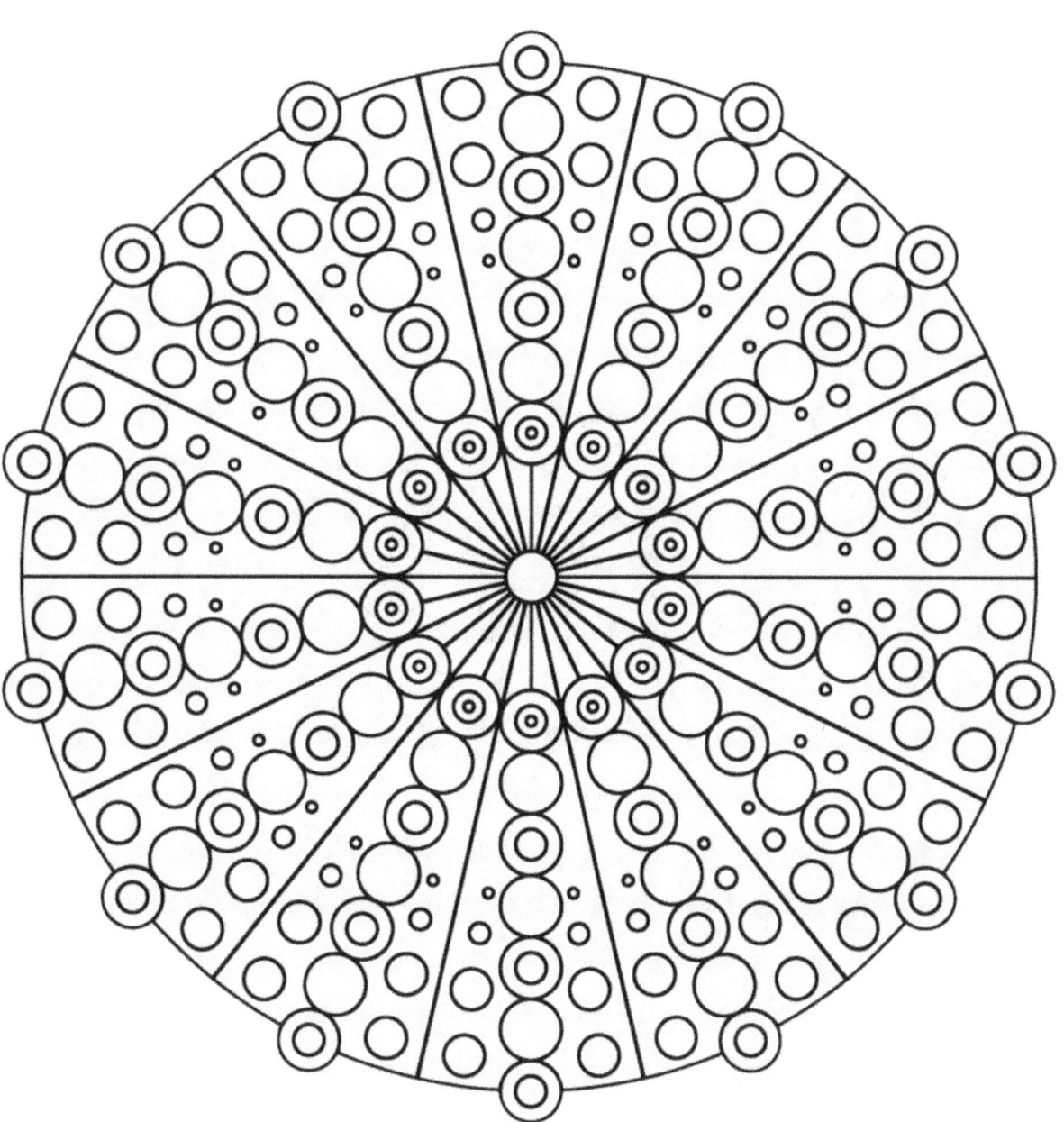

Your life is what your thoughts make of it!

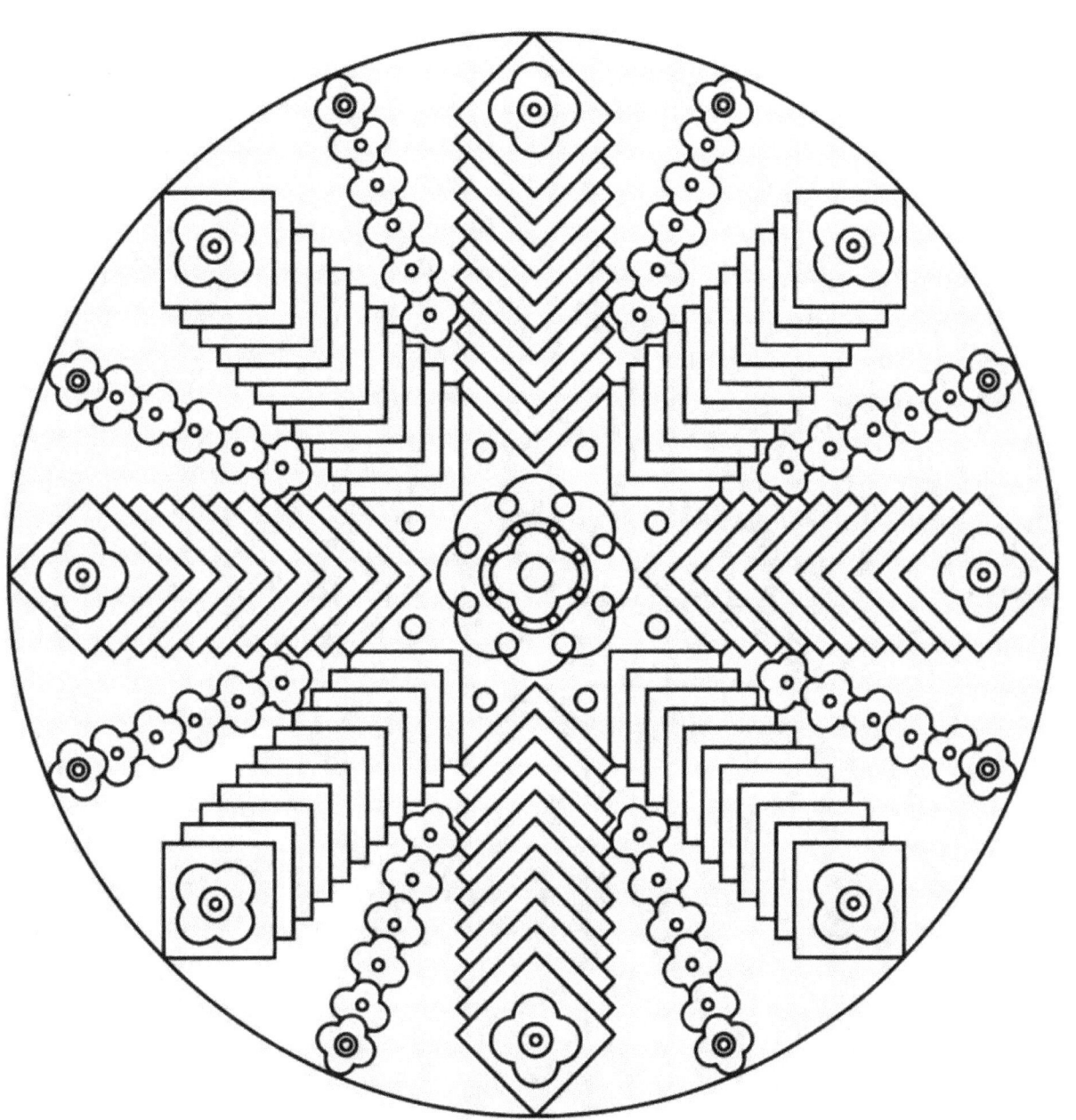

Broken crayons still color!

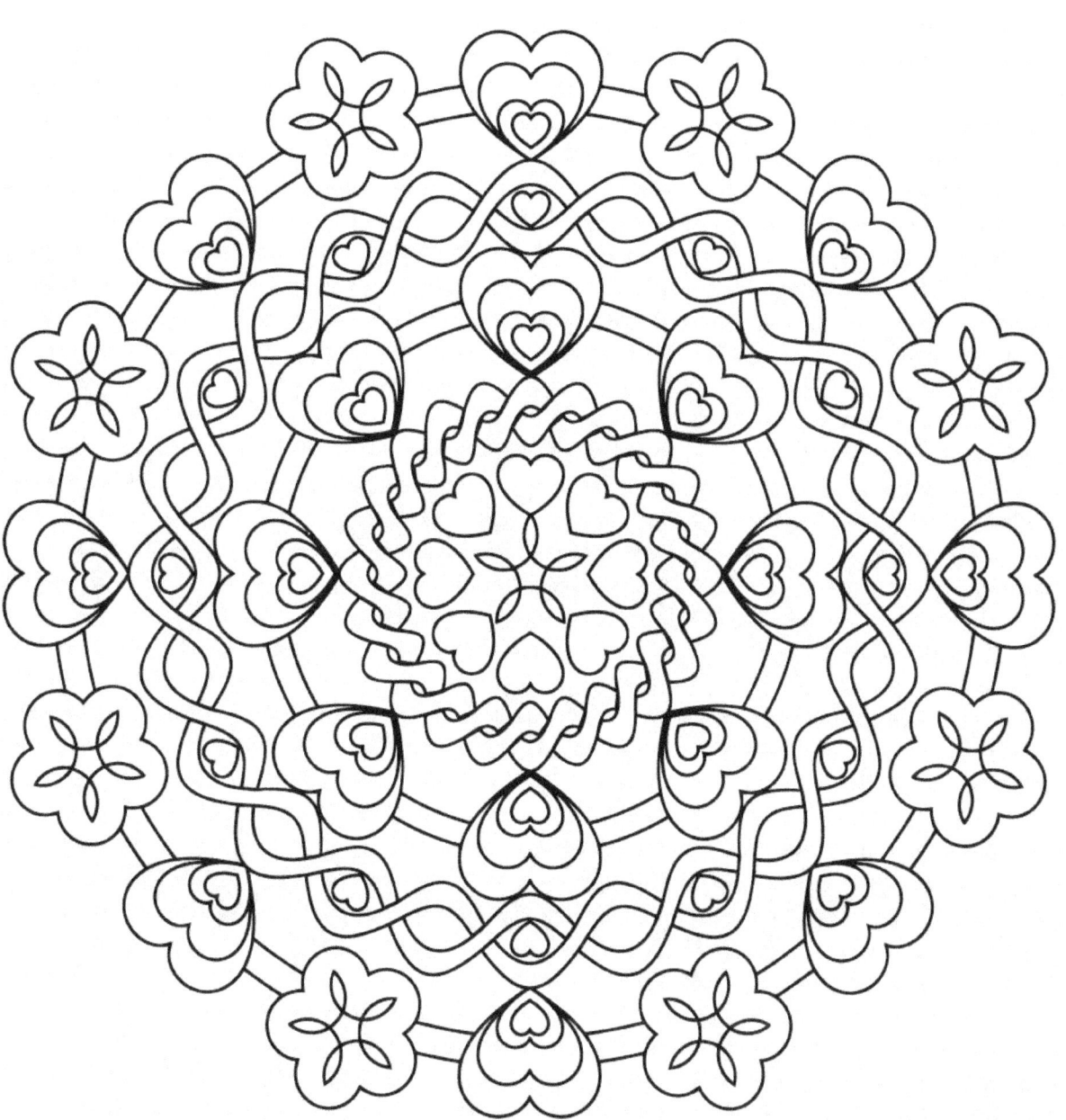

Collect moments, not things.

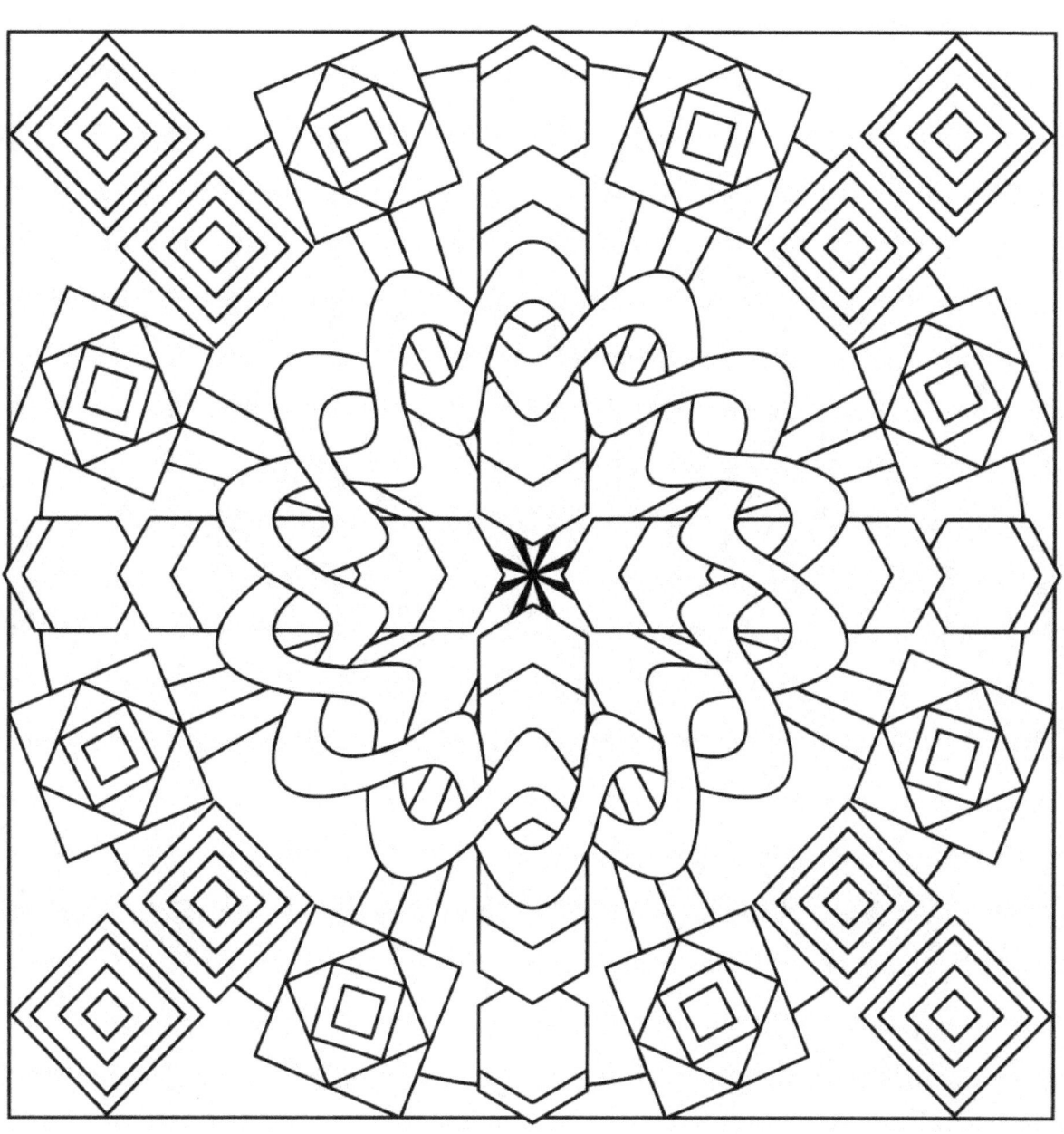

*Don't look back, you're
not going that way!*

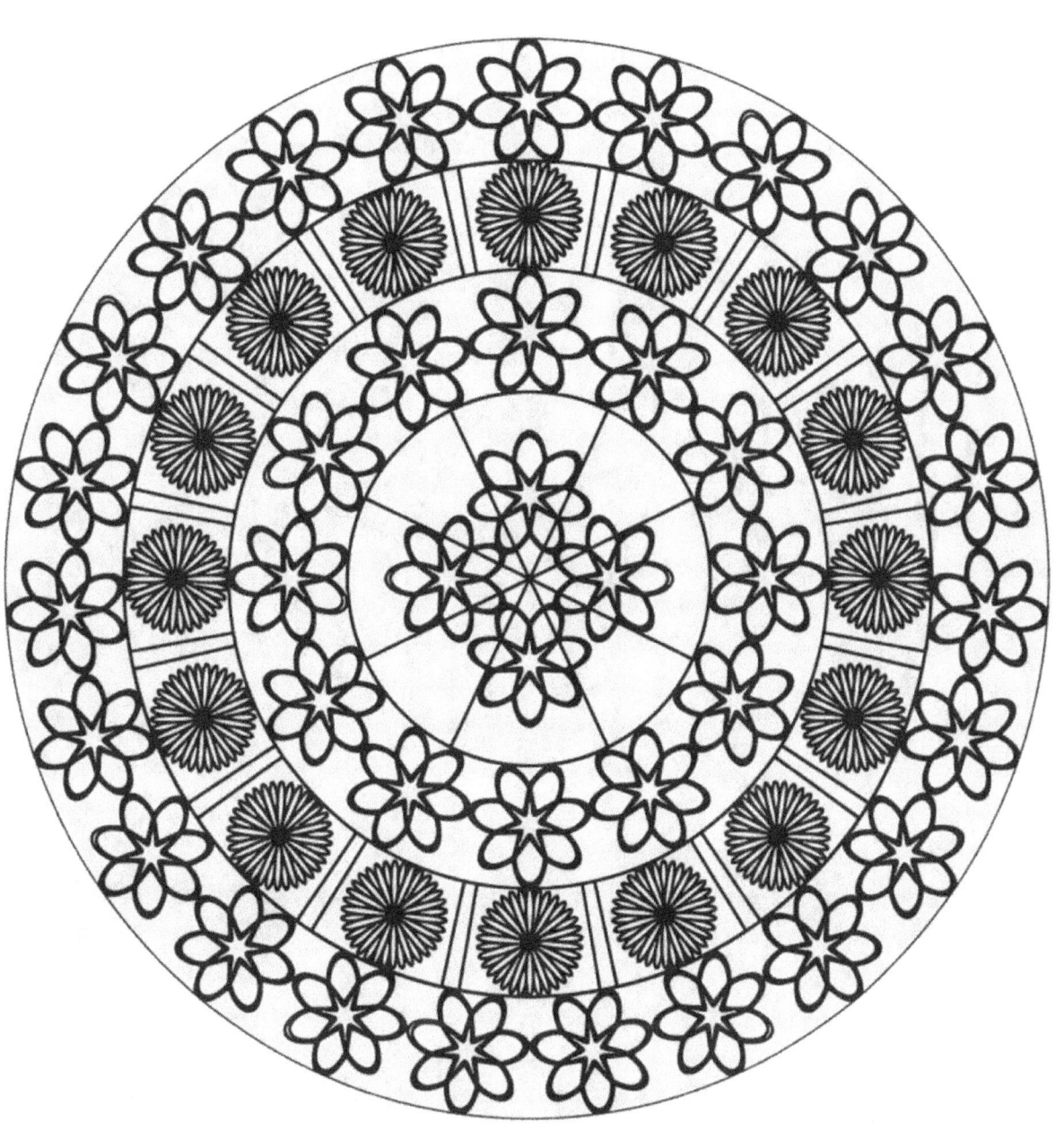

Color outside the lines!

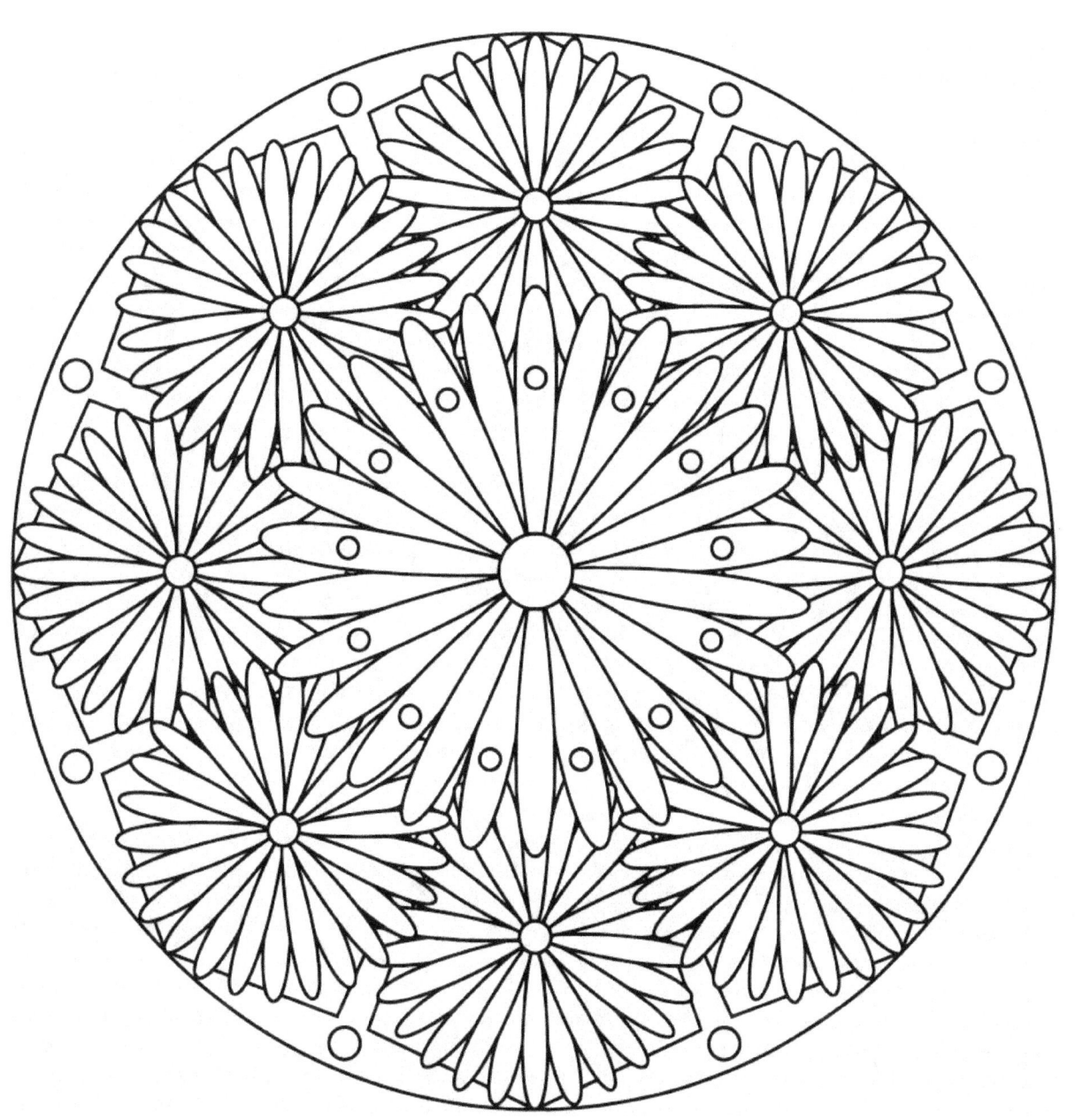

Live everyday of your life
to its fullest!

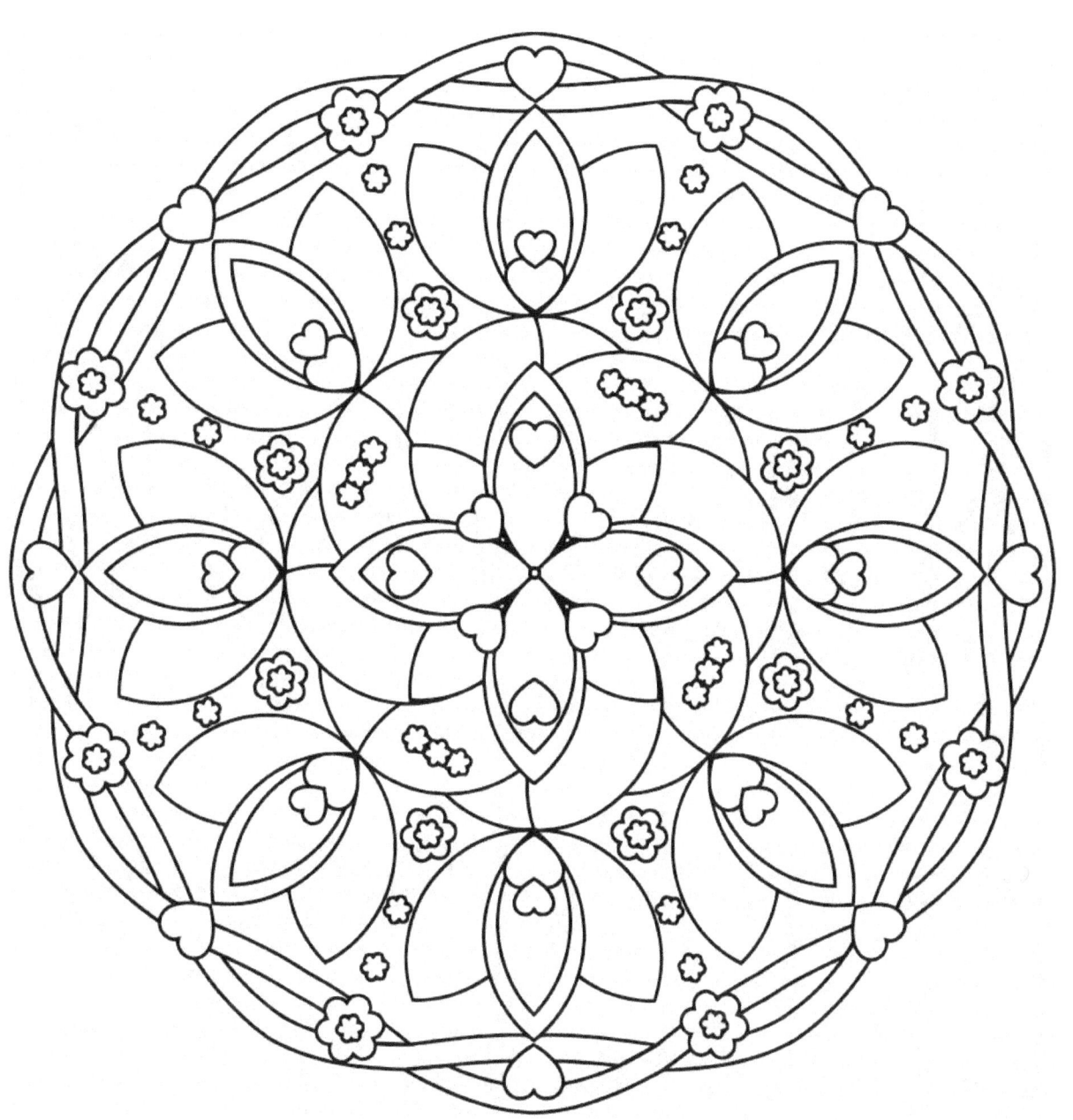

Being happy doesn't mean
that everything is perfect.
It means that you've
decided to look beyond
the imperfections.

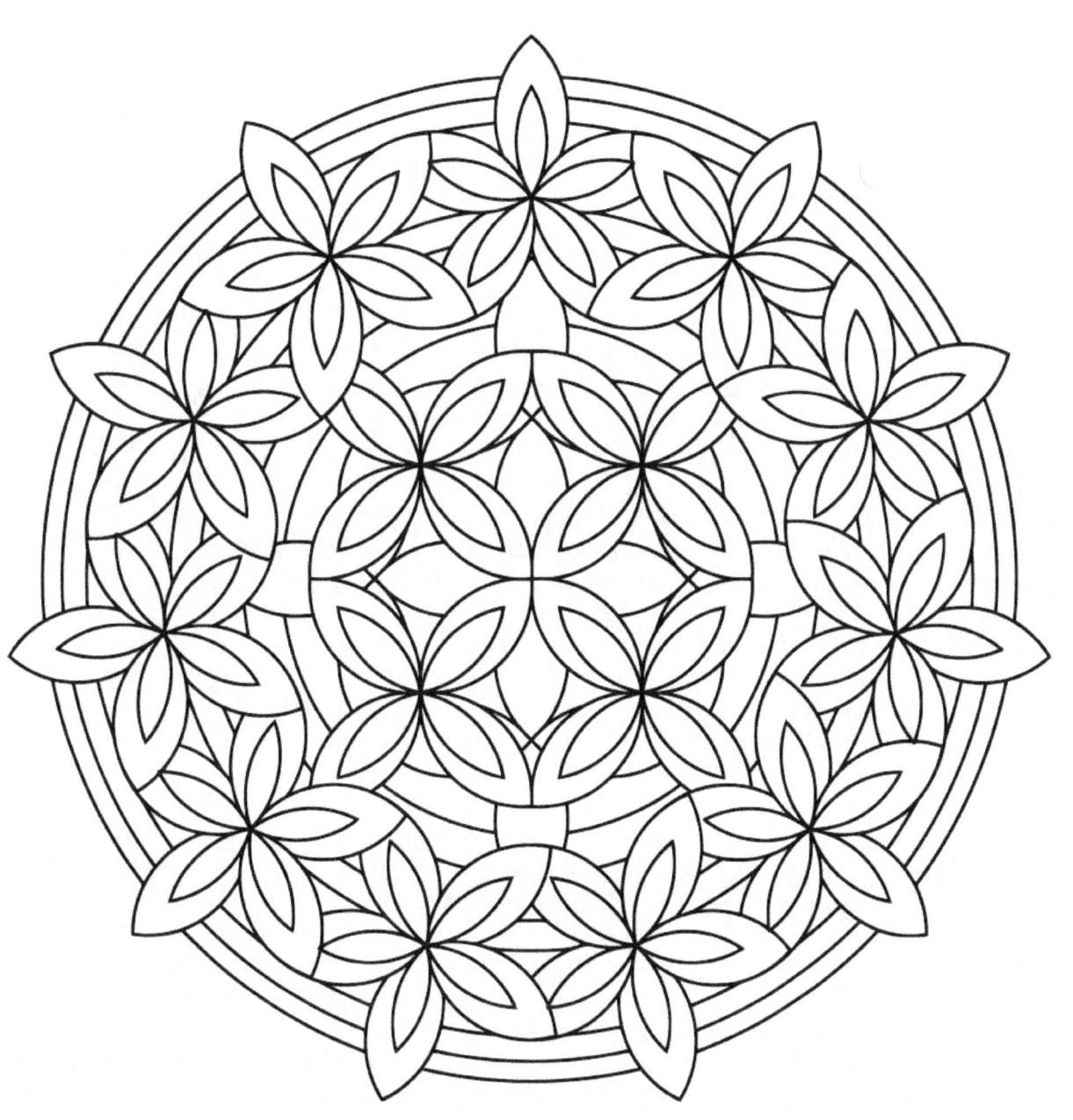

If it doesn't challenge you,
it won't change you.

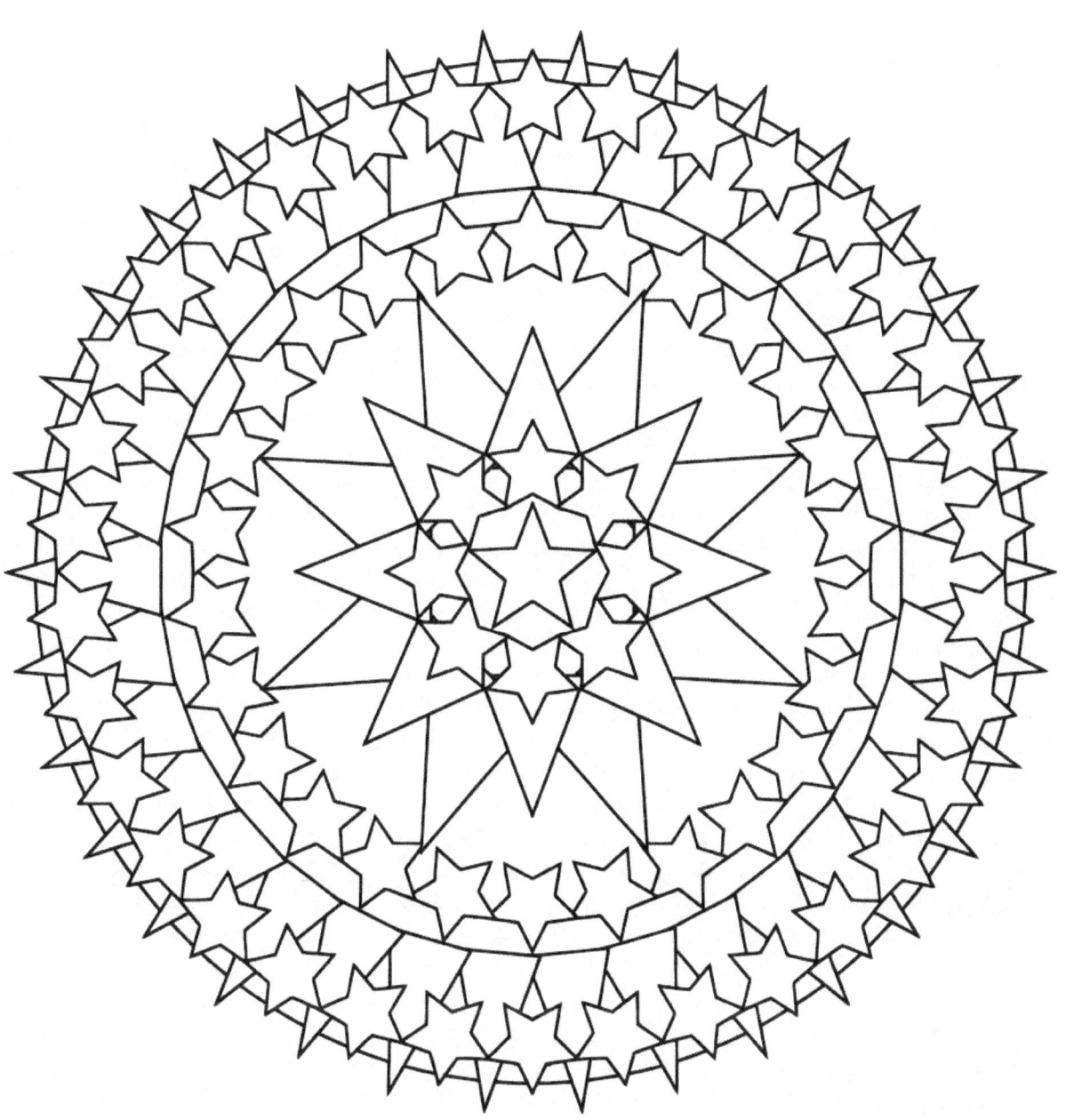

Keep going, you are nearly there!

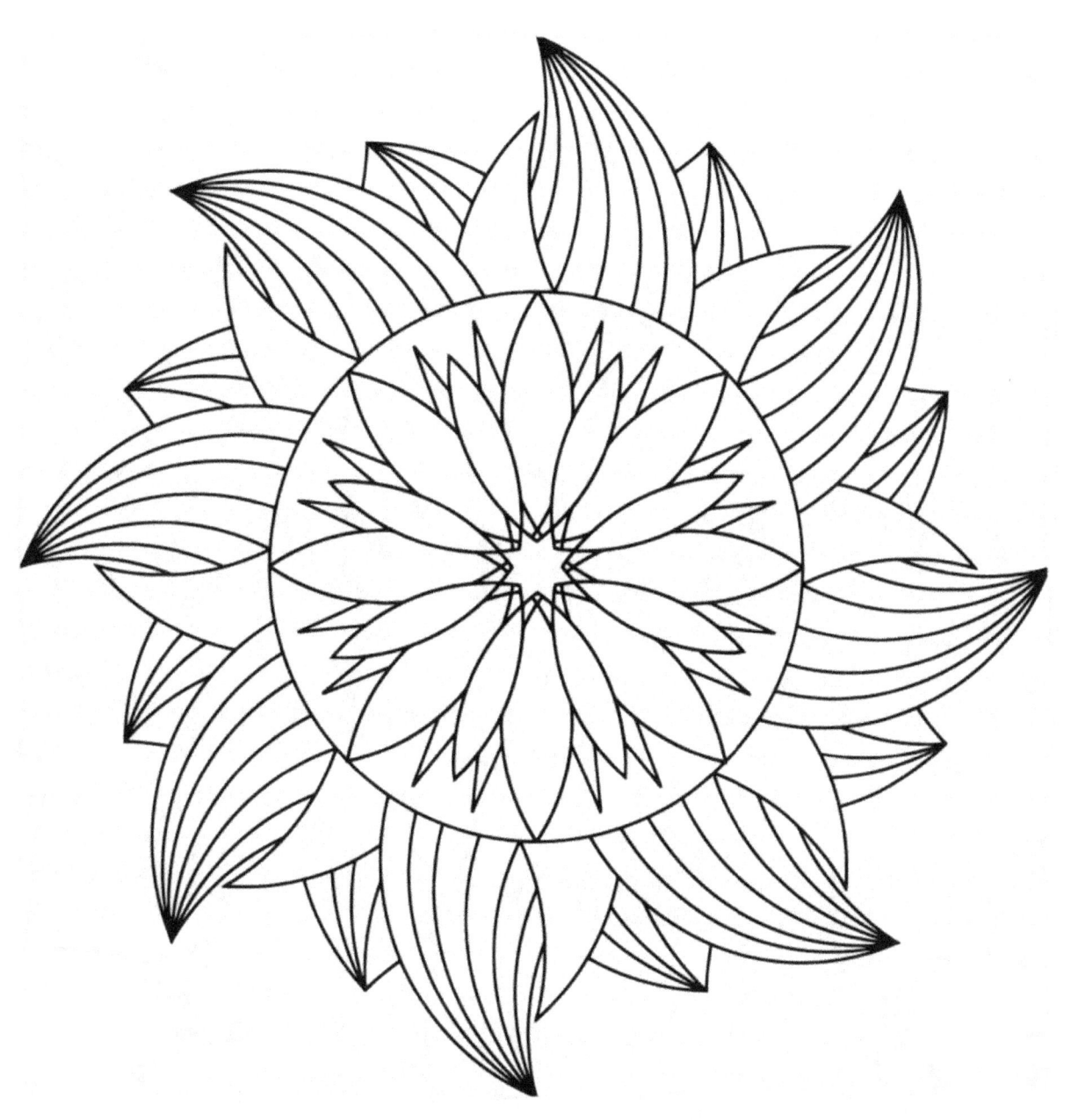

Open your mind and heart to new things!

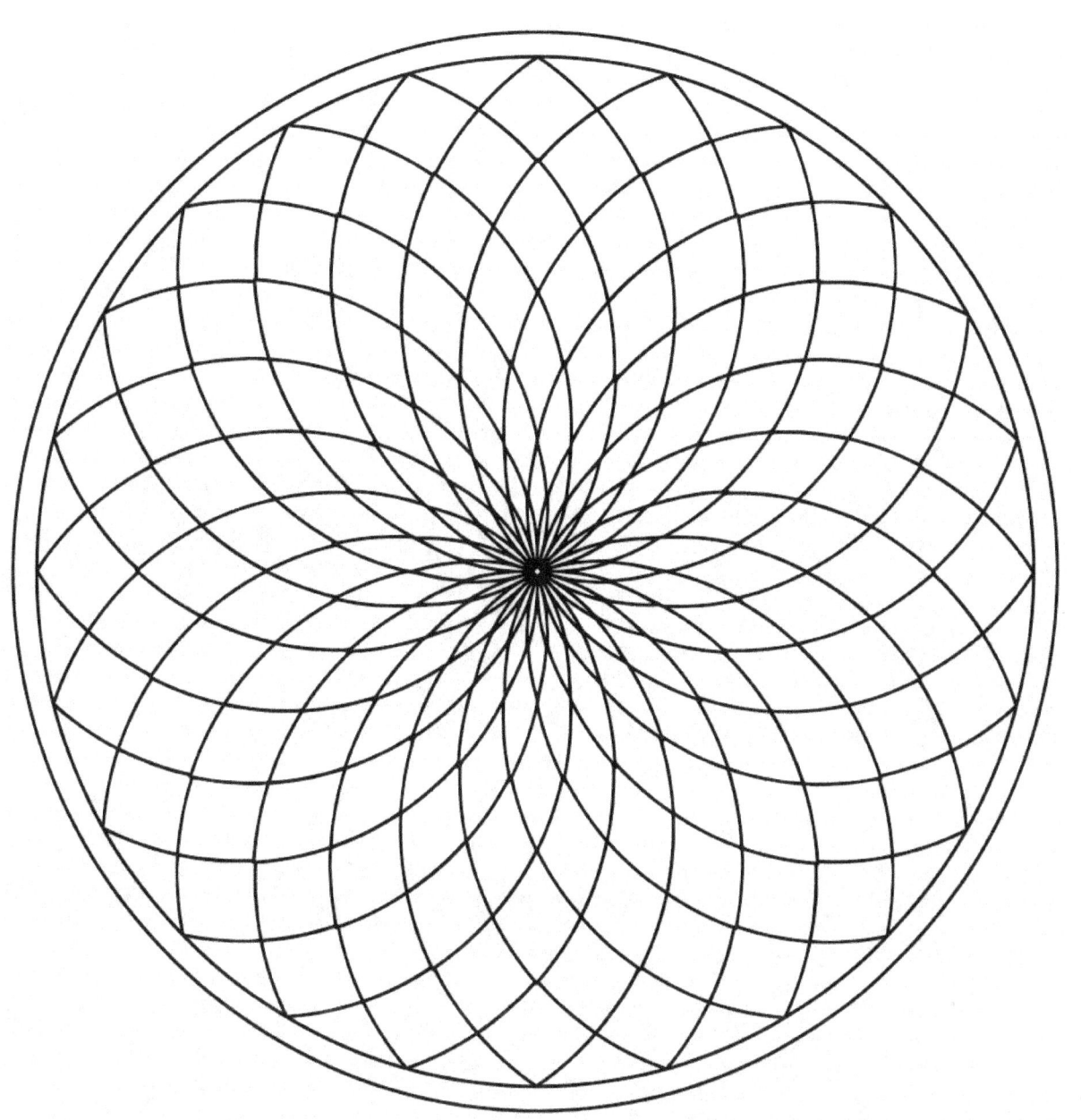

*Don't ruin a good today,
because of a bad
yesterday.*

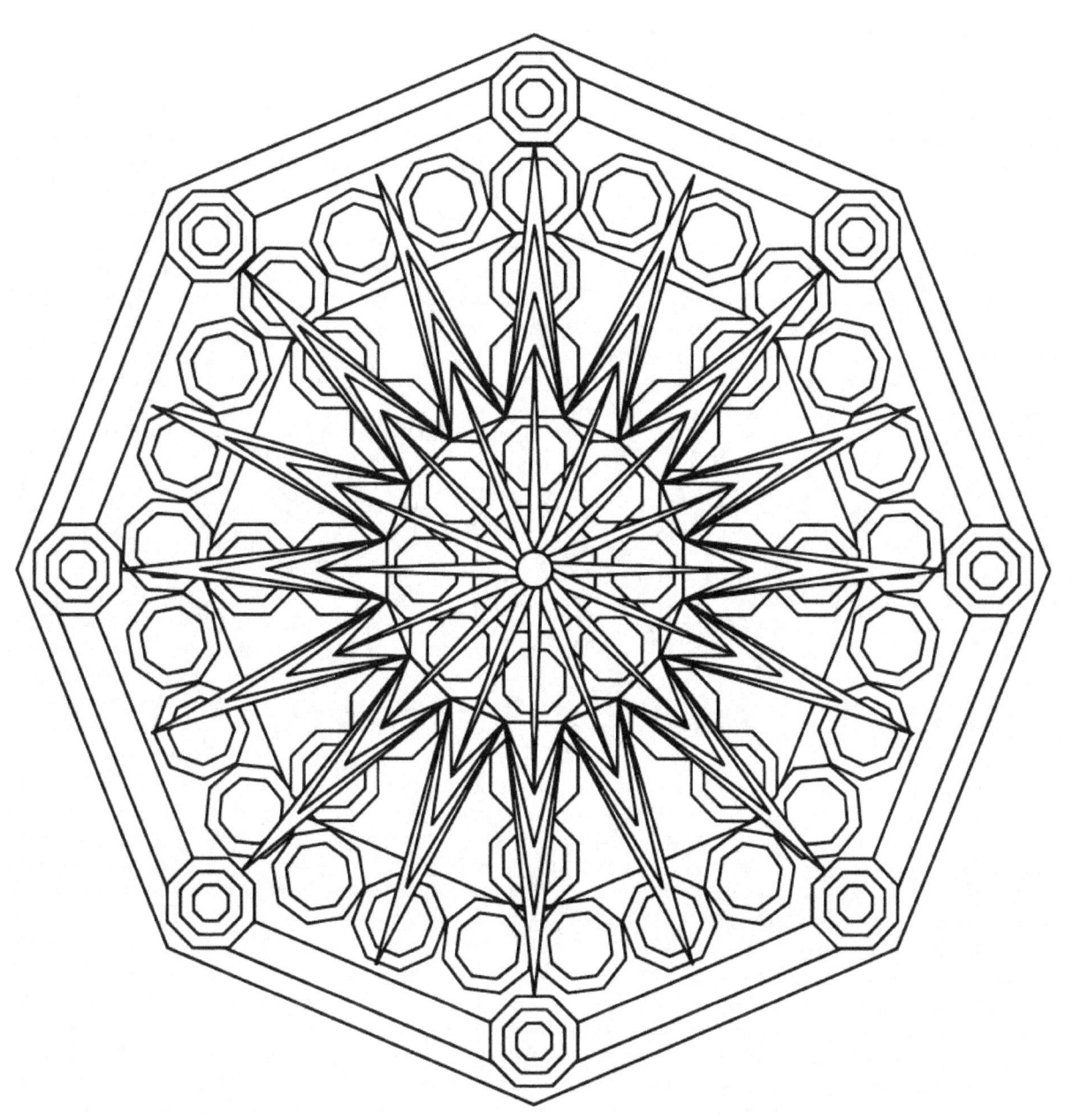

"Be helpful.
When you see a person
without a smile,
give them yours."

Zig Ziglar

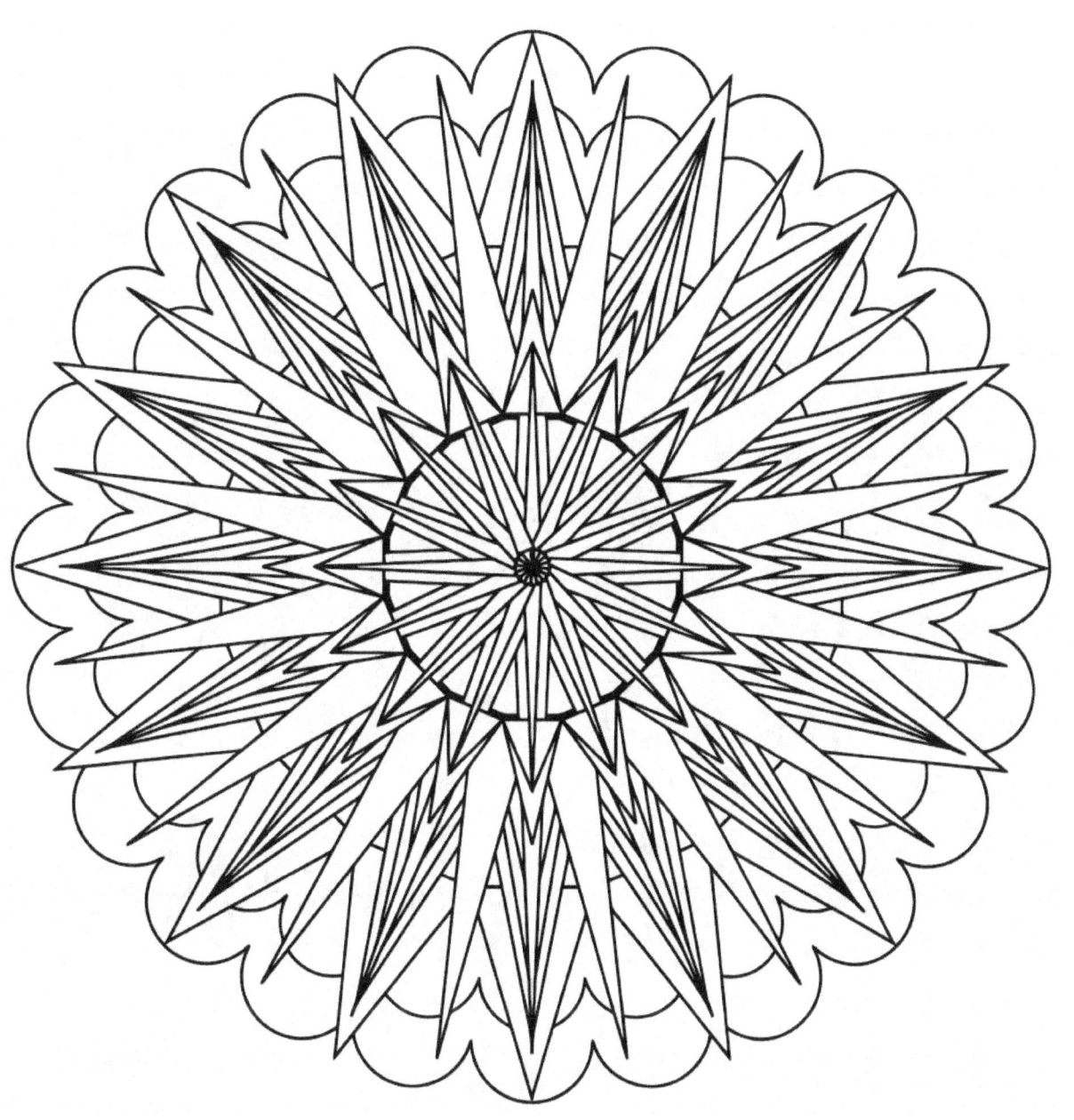

Stay In Touch & Explore More!

I hope you have enjoyed coloring this book and ask if you would please take just a moment to leave an honest review of my coloring book either on Etsy or Amazon.

I would also like to invite you to check out all of my Adult Coloring Books that are available as a paperback from Amazon here: https://amzn.to/2OK28P6 or as a PDF Digital download from my Etsy store here: https://www.etsy.com/au/shop/ColorYourWayToHappy

I love being creative and with over 40 books published so far, I'm always adding new books each month so be sure to check back and see if there's something you like.

Alternatively, if you would like to be kept up-to-date with new book releases and news please take the time to visit my Facebook page and feel free to let your friends and family know about my page too.

Don't forget to like and comment on my page and you're welcome to share your colored pages from my books there too!

Just go to: www.facebook.com/ColorYourWayToHappy

Thanks again and remember to have fun and go 'Color Your Way To Happy'!

Nerine ☺

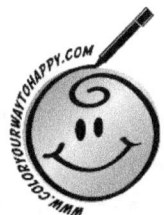

www.ingramcontent.com/pod-product-compliance
Lightning Source LLC
Chambersburg PA
CBHW082302200526
45168CB00017B/2748